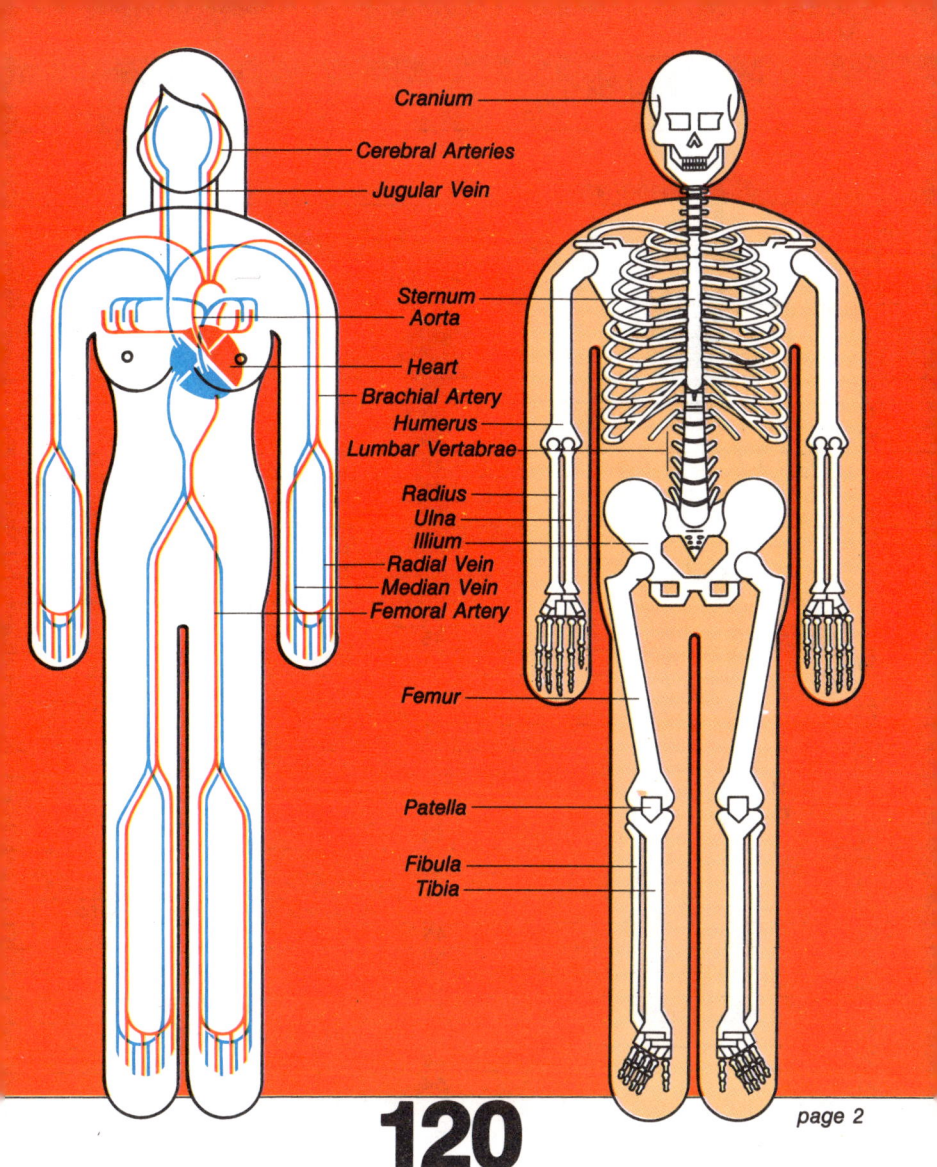

Cranium
Cerebral Arteries
Jugular Vein
Sternum
Aorta
Heart
Brachial Artery
Humerus
Lumbar Vertabrae
Radius
Ulna
Illium
Radial Vein
Median Vein
Femoral Artery
Femur
Patella
Fibula
Tibia

page 2

120
of the most common
DIAGNOSTIC TESTS

32
page 60

of the most common
SURGICAL PROCEDURES

74
page 94

of the most common
QUESTIONS & ANSWERS

Choosing a Doctor
What to do if surgery has been recommended
Hospitals
In the Hospital
Patient's Rights
Patient Responsibilities
Health Information
Insurance
Costs
Emergencies

Y0-DVF-640

Each patient carries his own doctor inside him. They came to us not knowing that truth. We are at our best when we give the doctor who resides within each patient a chance to go to work.

Albert Schweitzer

DIAGNOSTIC TESTS

- **1 ABDOMINAL ULTRASOUND**
  - ABG's — **5**
- **2 AIDS**
- **3 ALCOHOL**
- **4 AMNIOCENTESIS**
- **5 ARTERIAL BLOOD GASES**
- **6 ARTHROCENTESIS**
- **7 BARIUM ENEMA**
- **8 BARIUM SWALLOW**
- **9 BILIRUBIN**
  - Blood Gases — **5**
- **10 BLOOD PRESSURE**

11	**COMPLETE BLOOD COUNT**	**37**	**LIPASE**
12	**ACID PHOSPHATASE**	**38**	**LIPIDS**
13	**AIDS**	**39**	**MONONUCLEOSIS**
	AFP — **16,4**	**40**	**OSMOLALITY**
	A/G Ratio — **45**	**41**	**PARTIAL THROMBOPLASTIN TIME**
14	**ALCOHOL**	**42**	**PHOSPHORUS**
15	**ALKALINE PHOSPHATASE**	**43**	**PHENYLKETONURIA**
16	**ALPHAFETOPROTEIN**		PKU Test — **43**
17	**AMYLASE**	**44**	**POTASSIUM**
18	**BILIRUBIN**	**45**	**PROTEIN ALBUMIN/GLOBULIN RATIO**
	Blood Sugar — **30**	**46**	**PROTHROMBIN TIME**
19	**BLOOD TYPE & CROSS MATCH**		Pro Time — **46**
	Blood Urea Nitrogen — **20**		PT — **46**
20	**BUN**		PTT — **41**
21	**CALCIUM**		Red Blood Cell Count — **11**
22	**CARCINOEMBRYONIC ANTIGEN**		Red Blood Cell Differential — **11**
	CBC — **11**		Red Blood Cell Indices — **11**
	CEA — **22**	**47**	**RHEUMATOID FACTOR**
23	**CHOLESTEROL**	**48**	**RUBELLA TITER**
	CK — **25**		Sed Rate — **27**
24	**COOMBS' TEST**		Serum Glutamic Oxaloacetic Transaminase — **49**
25	**CREATINE PHOSPHOKINASE**		Serum Glutamic Pyruvic Transaminase — **50**
26	**CREATININE**	**49**	**SGOT**
27	**ERYTHROCYTE SEDIMENTATION RATE**	**50**	**SGPT**
28	**FASTING BLOOD SUGAR**	**51**	**SICKLE CELL**
	FTA-ABS — **53**	**52**	**SODIUM**
29	**GASTRIN**		SMA, SMA-6, SMA-12 — See Blood Tests
30	**GLUCOSE**	**53**	**SYPHILIS**
31	**GLUCOSE TOLERANCE TEST**	**54**	**TAY SACHS**
	GTT — **31**		Thyroid Stimulating Hormone — **56**
	Guthrie Test — **43**	**55**	**THYROXINE**
32	**HEPATITIS**		TIBC — **33**
	Hemoglobin — **11**		Triglycerides — **90**
	Hematocrit — **11**	**56**	**TSH**
33	**IRON, TOTAL IRON BINDING CAPACITY**		T₄ — **55**
34	**KETONES**	**57**	**URIC ACID**
35	**LACTIC DEHYDROGENASE**	**58**	**VITAMIN B-12 & FOLIC ACID**
	LDH — **35**		VDRL — **53**
36	**LEAD**		White Blood Cell Count & Differential — **11**

- Bone Biopsy — **59**
- **59 BONE MARROW ASPIRATION**
- **60 BONE SCAN**
  - Brain Wave Test — **75**
- **61 BRONCHOSCOPY**
  - Cardiac Angiography — **62**
- **62 CARDIAC CATHETERIZATION**
- **63 CARDIAC ENZYMES**
- **64 CARDIAC SCAN**
  - Cardiogram — **74**
- **65 CAT SCAN**
  - Cervical Smear — **98**
- **66 CHEST X-RAY**
- **67 CHLAMYDIA**
  - Chromosome Analysis — **4**
- **68 COLONOSCOPY**
- **69 COLPOSCOPY**
  - Culdoscopy — **89**
- **70 CREATININE CLEARANCE**
- **71 CYSTOSCOPY**
- **72 DOPPLER ULTRASOUND**

73	ECHOCARDIOGRAM
	EEG—75
	EKG—76
74	ELECTROCARDIOGRAM
75	ELECTROENCEPHALOGRAM
76	ELECTROLYTES
77	ENDOSCOPIC RETROGRADE CHOLANGIOPANCREATOGRAPHY
	ERCP—77
	Esophagram—8
	Eye Test—120
	Exercise Tolerance Test—109
78	FETAL MONITORING
	Fetal Ultrasound—4,78
79	FUNDOSCOPY
	Gallbladder Series—97
80	GASTRIC ANALYSIS
81	GASTROSCOPY
82	GONORRHEA
83	HEARING TEST
84	HEPATITIS
85	HERPES SIMPLEX II
	Holter Monitor—74
86	HYSTEROSALPINGOGRAPHY
87	INTRAVENOUS CHOLANGIOGRAPHY
88	INTRAVENOUS PYELOGRAPHY
	IVC—87
	IVP—88
89	LAPAROSCOPY
90	LIPIDS
91	LIVER SCAN
92	LIVER FUNCTION TESTS
	Lower GI—7
	Lumbar Puncture—108
93	LUNG SCAN
94	MAMMOGRAPHY
	Non-Stress Test—78
95	NUCLEAR MAGNETIC RESONANCE
96	OCCULT BLOOD
	Ophthalmoscopy—79
97	ORAL CHOLECYSTOGRAM
	Oxytoxin Challenge Test—78
98	PAP SMEAR
99	PET SCAN
100	PLETHYSMOGRAPHY
101	PREGNANCY
	Proctosidmoidoscopy—107
	Pulmonary Angiography—62
102	PULMONARY FUNCTION TESTS
103	PULSE
	Pyelogram—88
104	RADIOACTIVE IODINE UPTAKE/THYROID SCAN
105	RENAL ANGIOGRAPHY
106	SEMEN ANALYSIS
107	SIGMOIDOSCOPY
	Sperm Count—106
108	SPINAL TAP
109	STRESS TEST
	Stool—96
	Synovial Fluid—6
110	SYPHILIS
	TB Test—116
111	TEMPERATURE
112	THERMOGRAPHY
113	THROAT CULTURE
114	THYROID FUNCTION TESTS
	Thyroid Scan—104
115	TONOMETRY
116	TUBERCULOSIS SKIN TEST
117	UPPER GI
118	URINE ANALYSIS
119	VENOGRAPHY
120	VISUAL ACUITY
	TERMS

DIAGNOSTIC TESTS

One hundred years ago, a doctor had little more to go on than the patient's description of symptoms and the evidence of his or her senses. Was the patient feverish, the pulse weak or fast, the abdomen swollen, the urine cloudy?

Direct personal contact with the patient is still the cornerstone of diagnosis, but today's doctor also has access to an amazing array of technology. Flexible fiberoptic tubes enable the doctor to see deep inside the body. Computers help assemble images of the brain, and ultrasound reveals the beating of an unborn baby's heart.

Because we feel that knowledge helps you ask your doctor the right questions and take a positive role in getting well, we have included descriptions of 120 medical tests. Some may be performed more frequently than others, but all are in common use in American hospitals and doctors' offices. We have tried to indicate why the test might be ordered, how it is usually performed and what it feels like. The exact procedure may vary from place to place. If your experience is different from what is described in this book, it does not mean that your care is bad. It is just another thing we hope you will feel confident discussing with your doctor.

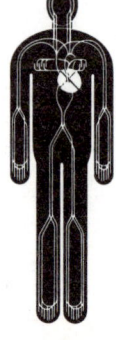

SYMBOLS & CHECKLIST

The illustrated figure to the left of an entry indicates at a glance either what organ is involved in a particular test, or where on the body the test takes place.

Invasive/Noninvasive. Tests that require probing, penetrating or injecting material into the body are invasive. They usually carry more risk and discomfort than noninvasive tests and they may require signing a consent form. **Cardiac catheterization** is invasive. An **electrocardiogram,** which uses sensors placed on the surface of the skin, is not. Though blood tests require a brief skin puncture, they are usually not considered invasive.

Pain. Keeping in mind that nothing is more personal and subjective than the experience of pain, we have tried to give you a sense of what to expect. Pain is rated on a scale from 0 to 5. Factored into the number is direct pain, as well as the discomfort you might feel from being in an awkward position or lying on a hard table for a long time. A chest x-ray is rated **0** for no pain. A blood test is rated **1**, very slight pain, and bone marrow aspiration is rated a **5**. Remember that terribly painful procedures are almost always done under anesthesia or sedation.

Consent. Before most invasive procedures you must sign a consent form. This form says that you have received a full explanation of the test, its procedures and potential risk. You don't have to sign the form until you are satisfied. The list of tests that require consent may vary from hospital to hospital. They generally include all endoscopic tests, tests where catheters are inserted, and tests where something is injected into the body.

Ask questions. Your doctor should be able to explain why the test is being ordered, what might be learned, and how the results will affect either diagnosis or treatment. When a complex test is ordered before a simple one, there may be a good reason, but you should have the doctor explain it to you. Lastly, do not be embarrassed to take notes. It can be a tense time and things get forgotten.

Follow directions. If a test requires that you fast, stop smoking, or stop medication, do what you are asked to do. Eating breakfast, for instance, before a glucose test could raise your blood sugar enough to make your doctor suspect diabetes and order more unnecessary tests.

Be alert and informed. Know what tests the doctor has ordered and how they are done. If you are in the hospital, make sure the people working on you are performing only the tests your doctor ordered. Make sure the people working on you know your correct name (first and last). Try to make sure that samples are labeled correctly.

Tell your doctor about:

Medication. Any drug you are taking including aspirin, laxatives, birth control pills, high blood pressure medication, thyroid medication, insulin, antibiotics, street drugs and alcohol, can influence the results of lab tests and lead your doctor to an incorrect diagnosis.

Allergies. People with allergies can have dangerous, even life-threatening reactions to certain tests, particularly x-rays that require an injection of an iodine based contrast dye. Take special care if you are allergic to iodine or seafood (which is high in iodine). The information should be on your chart and on a bracelet around your wrist.

Pregnancy. If you are pregnant or think you might be, your doctor must know. Certain tests should not be performed on pregnant women, and pregnancy can affect the results of many lab tests.

Athletics. People in training have different normal test values. For instance, a small amount of protein in the urine might be normal for a marathon runner but a sign of kidney disease in anyone else.

All illness. For reliable interpretation of test results and your own safety, your doctor must know about any kidney, heart, liver or lung disease, even if that is not what you are being tested for at the moment.

1 ABDOMINAL ULTRASOUND ABDOMINAL SONOGRAM

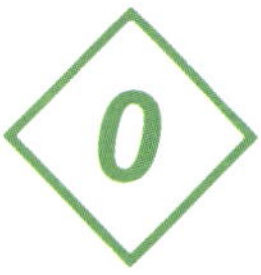

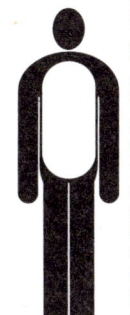

Ultrasound. It's the only thing submarines, porpoises and your internist have in common. In all 3 cases, the basic principle is the same. When high frequency sound waves (higher than can be heard by the human ear) are projected forward, they will continue moving until they bump into something, at which point a certain amount of sound bounces back. Submarine sonar operators use these echoes to measure the depth of the ocean floor and detect enemy mines; your doctor may use them to find gallstones.

In medical ultrasound, high frequency sound waves are emitted in regular pulses by a handheld instrument called a *transducer* that is moved across a part of your body. The transducer also receives the reflected sound waves, which are translated into electrical signals. An analysis of the *time* the pulse takes to bounce back can reveal the location of internal organs. Because tissues of varying densities reflect sound differently, the *amplitude* of the returning sound waves helps indicate tissue type. All this information is translated, often with computer enhancement, into black and white images on a TV monitor. These are then photographed for a permanent record. Most scans today visualize a two-dimensional cross section or slice of the body. However, some sophisticated *real time* ultrasound scanners send out rapid multiple pulses in a strict sequence that can be turned into moving images that show the heart in action, or the fetus moving in the womb.

Compared to the other imaging techniques in use—**CAT Scans, Nuclear Scans, X-Rays, Endoscopy**— ultrasound has a lot going for it. It is quick, fairly available and less expensive than any of the above, except for conventional x-rays. It is also non-invasive, painless and doesn't require contrast dye that can cause nausea or allergic reactions. But by far, its biggest advantage is that it doesn't expose the patient or the medical staff to radiation. Though numerous studies are now being done, no one during the last 30 years has been able to detect any long-or short-term side effects. It seems to be perfectly safe.

Nothing, however, is perfect. Ultrasound cannot penetrate bone or gas-filled spaces, so it is not useful in diagnosing problems in the skull, lungs, intestine or bowel. It also does not work well on obese patients or patients with bandages or large scars on the abdomen. Although it is more commonly available in hospitals than **CAT Scans** or **Nuclear Scans**, good results are more dependent on a skilled operator than they are in either of the other two studies.

The abdominal scan is one of the most common ultrasound studies, allowing an evaluation of almost all the abdominal organs, including the gallbladder, liver, spleen, lymph nodes and pancreas. It is fast becoming the test of choice in diagnosing gallstones, replacing more unpleasant and time-consuming tests like **Oral Cholecystogram** and **Intravenous Cholecystogram.** It is also the test of choice when trying to differentiate between solid masses and fluid-filled cystic masses in the liver, pancreas or elsewhere in the abdomen. Ultrasound is slowly replacing x-rays as a guiding system for doctors trying to find the best site for biopsy, and is now being used to detect abdominal injury in trauma victims. While there are certainly situations where a **CAT** scan or nuclear scan can reveal much more detailed information, many doctors now start the diagnostic process with ultrasound, moving on to more expensive and invasive means only when necessary.

For the average abdominal scan, little advance preparation is necessary. On rare occasions, you may be given a laxative or enema to clear the bowel of gas, and if you are going in for a gallbladder study, you may be asked to fast for 8-12 hours beforehand. (The gallbladder empties itself of bile and shrinks right after you have eaten. If you don't eat for a while, the gallbladder refills and is more easily visualized.)

If your personal physician doesn't have the equipment for abdominal ultrasound, and chances are he or she does not, you go to the radiology or ultrasound department of a hospital where you change into a loose gown. While you lie on your back on the examining table, a technician coats your abdomen with mineral oil. The liquid is a good sound conductor and allows the transducer to move freely over the surface of the skin. The technician or radiologist then takes the transducer—it looks like a microphone—and slides it back and forth across your abdomen. This is absolutely painless.

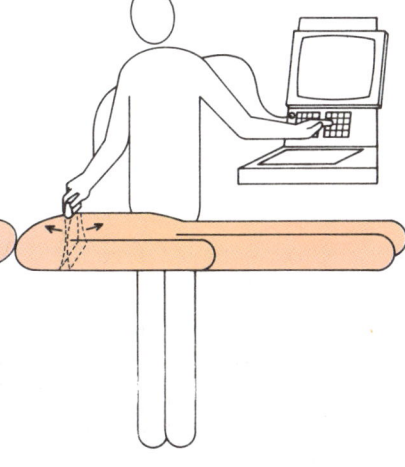

Ultrasound equipment varies from hospital to hospital. Some transducers may be attached to display and decoding machinery by a thin cable. Others are attached to the flexible metal arm of a large ceiling or wall-mounted console. In any event, the information is transmitted, projected and then recorded on video tape, polaroid film or heat-sensitive paper. The doctor will do a preliminary reading of the images while you are still on the table. If they turned out well, your abdomen is cleaned and you are allowed to leave. Though the picture can be examined immediately, a full report from the radiologist may take a day or so to get to your own personal physician.

Ultrasound is not limited to abdominal use. **Doppler Ultrasound** is used to evaluate blood flow in arteries and veins. **Echocardiography** has become a routine ultrasound study of the heart. And ultrasound monitoring of the fetus inside the mother's uterus has had vast influence on the contemporary practice of obstetrics. Ultrasound is also becoming increasingly popular in the evaluation of abnormal growths on small, difficult-to-image organs like the thyroid gland and the testicles.

You may also encounter *pelvic ultrasound,* used to visualize the kidneys, bladder and female reproductive organs. The procedure is only slightly different from an abdominal scan. You will be asked to drink several glasses of water before the exam and to hold your urine until the scanning is over. A full bladder helps sound wave conduction and also helps displace the bowel from the pelvic cavity, where it interferes with effective imaging. If the kidneys are being studied, you will be asked to lay on your stomach and the transducer will be moved across your back.

2 AIDS ACQUIRED IMMUNE DEFICIENCY SYNDROME

There is no one specific test to diagnose AIDS. Though AIDS is probably caused by a viral agent, it is not so much a separate disease,

as a syndrome in which a devastating breakdown of the immune system leaves the body susceptible to a series of other deadly diseases that most people never contract. Two diseases in particular are the most common causes of death in AIDS victims: *Kaposi's sarcoma,* an obscure cancer; and *Pneumocystis Carinii pneumonia*—a pneumonia not caused by the usual viral or bacterial agents and practically unheard of in the general population.

A diagnosis of AIDS is generally made by diagnosing one of the above diseases after taking a careful medical history and performing a thorough physical exam. Kaposi's sarcoma (KS) is identified by biopsying (taking a tissue sample) and examining microscopically either a lymph node or a tumor. Tumors are usually found on the skin; however, KS tumors can also be internal. The pneumonia can only be diagnosed by biopsying a small sample of lung tissue, which must be done as part of **Bronchoscopy.**

There are also several complex blood tests that analyze the levels of certain cells of the immune system, called *T-helper cells* and *T-suppressor cells.* A healthy person has more helper cells than suppressor cells, but for AIDS victims, the proportions may be reversed.

A commercial blood test kit was approved by the government in 1985, which tests the blood for antibodies to the virus suspected of causing AIDS. It was designed as a screening procedure for blood banks and was not intended for diagnostic use. It indicates only past exposure to the virus, not whether or not someone has AIDS now, or will ever contract it. (Current studies indicate that only 1-2 percent of all who test positive will get AIDS.) The test yields results in 4 hours and is relatively inexpensive. By the end of the year this screening test will probably be done on all blood donations and is expected to add several dollars to the price a hospitalized patient pays for a unit of blood.

As the blood screening test becomes more widely available in doctor's offices and community centers, the controversy grows over who should be tested. Many health professionals advise those in high risk groups (primarily gay men) not to get tested unless they are showing other symptoms or have had a relationship with a known victim. They maintain that a positive result really tells you nothing useful, while at the same time it may cause needless worry. The minority view, in favor of testing, maintains that it is better to know, to be carefully followed medically, and to be prepared to act immediately if and when a breakthrough in treatment comes along.

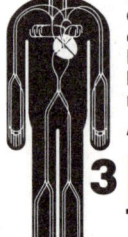

3 ALCOHOL

The alcohol test does not measure how much you have drunk, it measures the percentage of alcohol in your blood. It is this percentage, not

the actual volume of alcohol consumed, that determines how much function is impaired. Emergency room patients who are unconscious or acting strangely may be tested for alcohol in the blood, but the test is used much more frequently to evaluate the blood alcohol level of someone suspected of driving while intoxicated. In most states a blood level of 0.1 percent or more is legal proof of drunkenness. Anyone with a level of 0.25 percent approaches alcoholic stupor and someone with a blood alcohol level of 0.4 percent soon lapses into a coma which can be fatal.

Blood alcohol levels can also be measured by a breath test. You breathe into a machine that analyzes the last part of the breath called the *alveolar air.* If there is alcohol in the blood, it will be present as vapor in the exhaled air. Special fluids that change color in the presence of alcohol are exposed to the exhaled air inside the machine. The color change is measured photoelectrically and translated into a numerical result. Eating or drinking non-alcoholic substances after drinking will not alter the results.

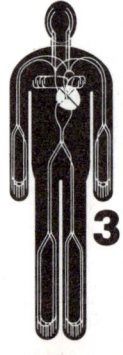

4 AMNIOCENTESIS

During pregnancy the fetus floats inside the uterus in a warm cushioning bath of amniotic fluid. This fluid contains cells shed by the fetus as it matures.

An analysis of the fluid and cells can yield valuable information about the fetus, including the presence of birth defects like *Down's syndrome* and *spina bifida,* metabolic disorders like Tay Sachs and *sickle cell anemia, and* overall fetal health, maturity and sex. During amniocentesis, 3-5 teaspoons of amniotic fluid are withdrawn from the uterus, usually between the 14th and 18th week of pregnancy when sufficient fluid is present to make the procedure safe, and yet when enough time remains to terminate the pregnancy within the legal time limit, should abnormalities be found.

Until recently the procedure was only offered in cases where there was a high risk of fetal abnormality—mother over 35, previous child with birth defects—or with mothers who have an underlying disease like high blood pressure or diabetes which might make her unable to carry the baby to term. But now a combination of advances, most notably in the ultrasound techniques that help the physician locate the fetus and placenta, have greatly reduced the risks associated with this procedure. As couples across the nation have fewer children and have them later in life, their concern naturally increases that everything will turn out just right. More and more, relief of maternal anxiety is considered justification for amniocentesis.

Amniocentesis is usually performed on an outpatient basis at a hospital or specially-equipped clinic. No special patient preparation is needed. Right before the procedure, you will be asked to urinate and a blood sample may be taken. You lie on your back on an examining table while the fetal heart rate is determined with a special stethoscope. Then the location of the fetus and placenta is determined by ultrasound. An oily lubricant is spread on your belly and the ultrasound transducer, which looks like a microphone, is passed over it. The doctor may press gently on your abdomen to shift the baby to a higher position.

Once fetal position is determined, the area right above the pubic bone is cleansed and may be draped with sterile cloth so that only a small part is visible. The skin and underlying muscle is numbed with an injection of local anesthetic. This stings like any needle would, but it doesn't last long. When the abdomen is numb, the doctor inserts a much longer needle through the skin, abdominal and uterine walls, into the amniotic cavity and withdraws a small amount of fluid. It is usual to feel pressure and perhaps some cramping while this is happening.

When the sampling is complete, the needle is withdrawn and a small bandage put over the puncture site. The fetal heart rate is assessed once again and you are allowed to rest. While you are resting, your pulse, temperature, blood pressure and any contractions you may have are noted. If you have RH negative blood and the father has RH positive blood, you may be given a gamma globulin shot. This is to ensure that in case the fetus has RH positive blood, there will be no adverse reaction between the fetus' blood and your blood. The shot is usually given in your behind and it hurts more than the test itself.

You should be able to leave the hospital and resume normal activity immediately. You will be advised to notify your doctor immediately if you have abdominal pain, more contractions than usual, a change in fetal activity, fever, vaginal drainage or bleeding.

A full analysis of the amniotic fluid assesses the following:

Genetic and chromosomal abnormalities. An examination of the chromosomes (where genetic information is stored) of cultured fetal cells can show whether or not the fetus has Down's syndrome, a severe form of mental retardation, and probably the most common birth defect, affecting 1 out of every 600-800 births. Incidence of Down's syndrome and other related types of genetic retardation increase with the age of the mother. In 1000 pregnant women, the incidence is: at age 25, 2; at 35, 5; at 40, 15.8. Certain other hereditary conditions like *muscular dystrophy* and *hemophilia* can also be detected by chromosome analysis.

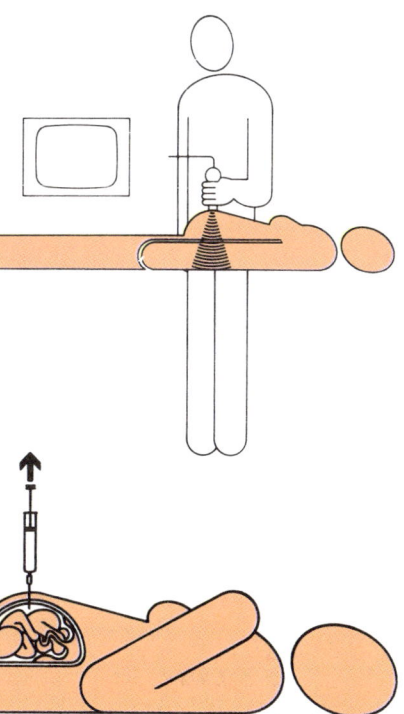

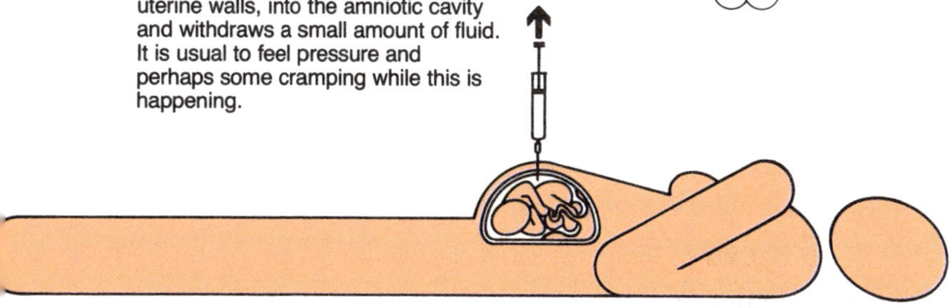

Metabolic disorders. There are several hundred genetically determined disorders of the metabolism, but so far, only a few of them can be detected by culturing the cells of the fetus. They include *sickle cell anemia* and *Tay Sachs*. Carrier status for both these diseases can be screened for in the parents before conception. But the screening only yields a statistical likelihood. Some couples may decide to risk pregnancy anyway in the hope that amniocentesis will tell them that their child will be healthy.

Neural tube defects. The most common neural tube defect is *spina bifida*, a condition where the fetal spinal column fails to develop properly. Children affected with spina bifida are frequently stillborn or die soon after birth. Those who survive may be retarded and partially paralyzed. To detect a fetus with a neural tube defect, the amniotic fluid is tested for alphafetoprotein (AFP), one of the main components of fetal blood. When there is incomplete closure of the spinal column, AFP leaks into the amniotic fluid. These high levels can be detected in the lab. Approximately 1 out of every 2000 babies is born with spina bifida. This goes up to 1 in 40 if the mother has already given birth to one child with spina bifida.

Fetal maturity. Fetal maturity is commonly a concern in high risk pregnancies when some underlying medical problems, like multiple births, diabetes or severe hypertension, exist, making it more likely that the mother may not be able to safely carry the child to term. In these cases, where an obstetrician is considering inducing labor or when a cesarean delivery may be necessary, it is important to know how mature the fetus is, or in other words, what its chances for survival are if born early. Several different tests are done on the amniotic fluid, the most important, the *L/S ratio*, measures fetal lung maturity. In this case, amniocentesis is often done much later in pregnancy, during or after the 35th week.

While it is true that amniocentesis is a relatively safe procedure, and is now performed routinely across the nation, there are risks. These include infection, bleeding, and in about 1 in 300 cases, miscarriage. On the other hand, 1 in 300 is also about the same chance a woman of 35 has of having a baby with Down's syndrome. Another thing to consider is that for some parts of the test, including chromosome analysis, results are not available for 2-4 weeks, when abortion is more complicated, both medically and psychologically. The decision to have amniocentesis should be carefully discussed by the couple and with their doctor. In general, it is recommended for women over 35, women who have previously given birth to a child with birth defects and when one or both parents have a genetic disease or a history of it. The test is not usually recommended for couples who would not consider having a therapeutic abortion if the results indicated a fetus with severe birth defects.

Chorionic villi sampling (CVI) is a new technique for detection of fetal birth defects that many believe will eventually replace amniocentesis. It is currently undergoing study at hospitals across the nation. The chief advantage of the new method is speed. Unlike amniocentesis, performed during the 16th week of pregnancy, CVI is usually performed in the 9th or 10th week. Some results, including whether the fetus has Down's syndrome, are available within 2 days. A full report takes 2 weeks, about as long as a full report from amniocentesis. If the results lead the parents to opt for therapeutic abortion, they can do so earlier in the pregnancy, when the procedure is safer and when it is more easily accepted psychologically. The procedure itself is relatively painless and is usually done without anesthesia. A small catheter or tube is guided by ultrasound into the uterus, until it comes in contact with the *chorion*, a membrane that surrounds the fetus and will later develop into the *placenta*. Fine filaments of tissue, the *villi*, protrude from the membrane. A few of these are aspirated through the catheter and then examined in the lab. Studies are not yet complete, but preliminary results suggest a miscarriage rate of between 1 and 2 percent, slightly higher than the miscarriage rate for amniocentesis which is generally thought to be between 2/3 and 1/2 of 1 percent.

5 ARTERIAL BLOOD GASES

Measures the amount of oxygen and carbon dioxide dissolved in the blood as well as the blood's pH (degree of acidity). Blood moves constantly through the lungs; with each breath it gives up poisonous carbon dioxide and takes in oxygen. Therefore, a measure of these gases in the blood is a good indication of how well the lung is functioning, and, to a lesser extent, the ability of the heart to pump blood through the lungs.

Although the test is not truly painful, it does hurt more than a standard blood test. The blood gas sample must be fresh from the heart and lungs, so the sample is taken from an artery. All other blood tests rely on a sample taken from a vein, but venous blood has already made a long trip through the body and is oxygen depleted. Arteries are slightly deeper than veins and harder to locate by sight. In addition to having to go a bit deeper under the skin, there is also a greater chance that the technician or doctor taking the sample will have to prick you several times to find an artery. The radial artery in the wrist is used most frequently, followed by the brachial artery on the inner surface of the elbow. In rare circumstances, the femoral artery in the groin is used.

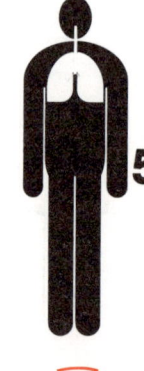

The technician uses a special oil-coated syringe which prevents any room air from contaminating the blood sample. After the needle is withdrawn, direct pressure should be applied to the puncture wound for several minutes. The sample is usually rushed to the lab for immediate analysis. If this is impossible, the sample is packed in ice to keep it stable.

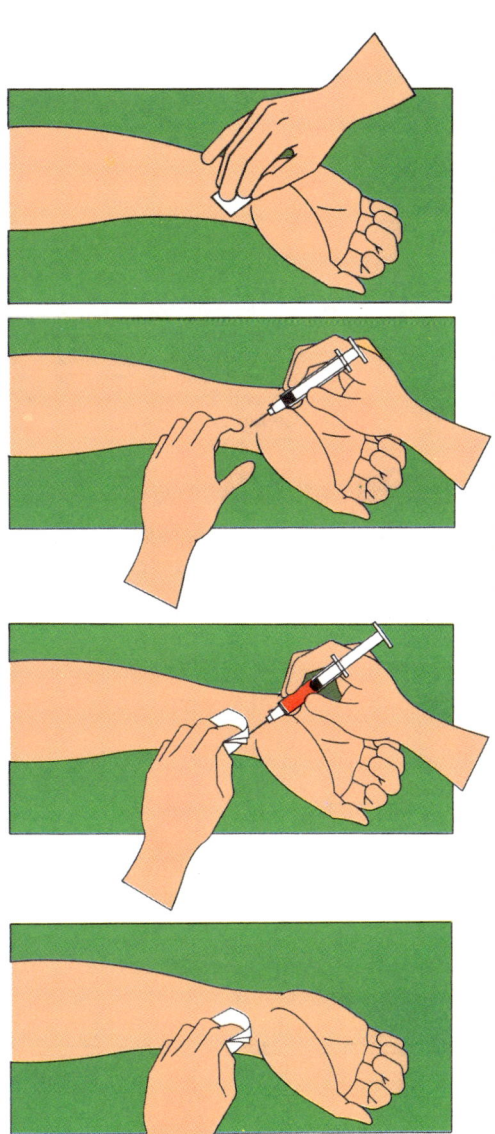

The test is done whenever serious lung disease or malfunction is suspected, as in *pneumonia, emphysema, pulmonary embolism* (blood clot in the lung) or *congestive heart failure* (fluid in the lungs). In these cases it is often performed in conjunction with **PULMONARY FUNCTION TESTS.** The test may also be administered to patients with severe uncontrolled *diabetes*. Their blood may become too acidic, a dangerous condition that can be detected by analyzing blood pH. Arterial blood gases are also measured before some surgeries, such as chest surgery, where the results can help determine the correct type of anesthesia. The test may then be repeated after surgery to evaluate how well the anesthesia was tolerated. The test is also used to evaluate victims of smoke inhalation and to screen miners, asbestos workers and others who are exposed to hazardous fumes and dust at the workplace.

Pulmonary Embolism. *A blockage in one of the arteries that bring blood from the heart to the lungs. Most originate from a blood clot in a deep vein in the leg. Part of the clot detaches from the vein wall, travels through the heart and lodges in the lungs. Lung tissue beyond that point can't exchange carbon dioxide for oxygen. This reduces the amount of oxygenated blood returning to the left side of the heart and puts an extra strain on the right side. Pulmonary embolism can be a complication of* thrombophlebitis *(vein inflammation) or lengthy surgery that is followed by prolonged bedrest. Massive embolism can cause collapse and death. Less severe cases may cause chest pain, breathlessness, faintness, bloody sputum or blueness around the lips.*

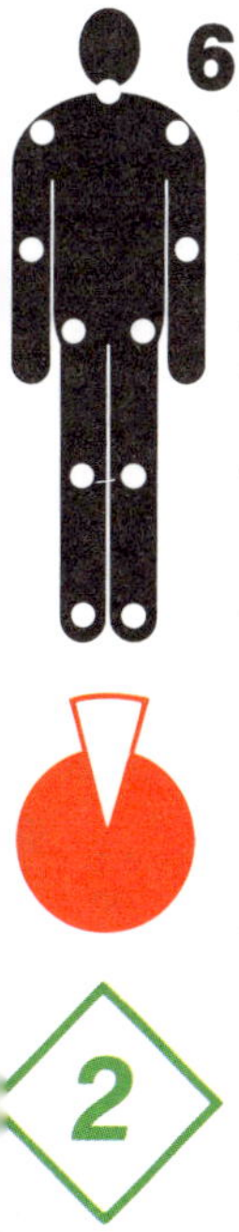

6 ARTHROCENTESIS SYNOVIAL FLUID

Within most joints there is a small amount of liquid (synovial fluid) that acts as a lubricant for surfaces that come in contact with each other

hundreds of times a day. Normally this is a clear fluid with a light yellow tint and the consistency of maple syrup. Swelling, pain or fever in a joint may be accompanied by changes in the synovial fluid. When attempting to diagnose arthritis or infection within the joint, your physician may want a sample of synovial fluid for study. The sample is most commonly taken from the knee, though shoulder, hip, elbow, wrist and ankle may also be sampled. The procedure lasts about 10 minutes and can be done in a doctor's office.

The knee is cleaned thoroughly, coated with iodine and covered with a cloth so only a small section of skin is exposed. You may be given a local anesthetic with a small needle, or the knee may be sprayed with a freezing substance which numbs the area. Then a longer needle is quickly inserted through the skin and into a joint cavity. Fluid is withdrawn. The needle is removed and pressure put on the puncture site. In some cases pressure or an elastic bandage will be applied, above and below the joint, to force fluid into an area where it can be collected. While some patients report that the procedure is painful, most find it merely uncomfortable and a bit disquieting to watch the long needle penetrate the joint. In some cases, where there is swelling and an excess of fluid due to inflammation or internal bleeding, the withdrawal of fluid may actually bring relief of pain. Typically, you can resume functioning immediately but with some care taken to avoid overexertion. You may be told to apply ice or an ace bandage. Watch for any signs of increased swelling, heat or pain at the site of the procedure and immediately report any symptoms to your doctor.

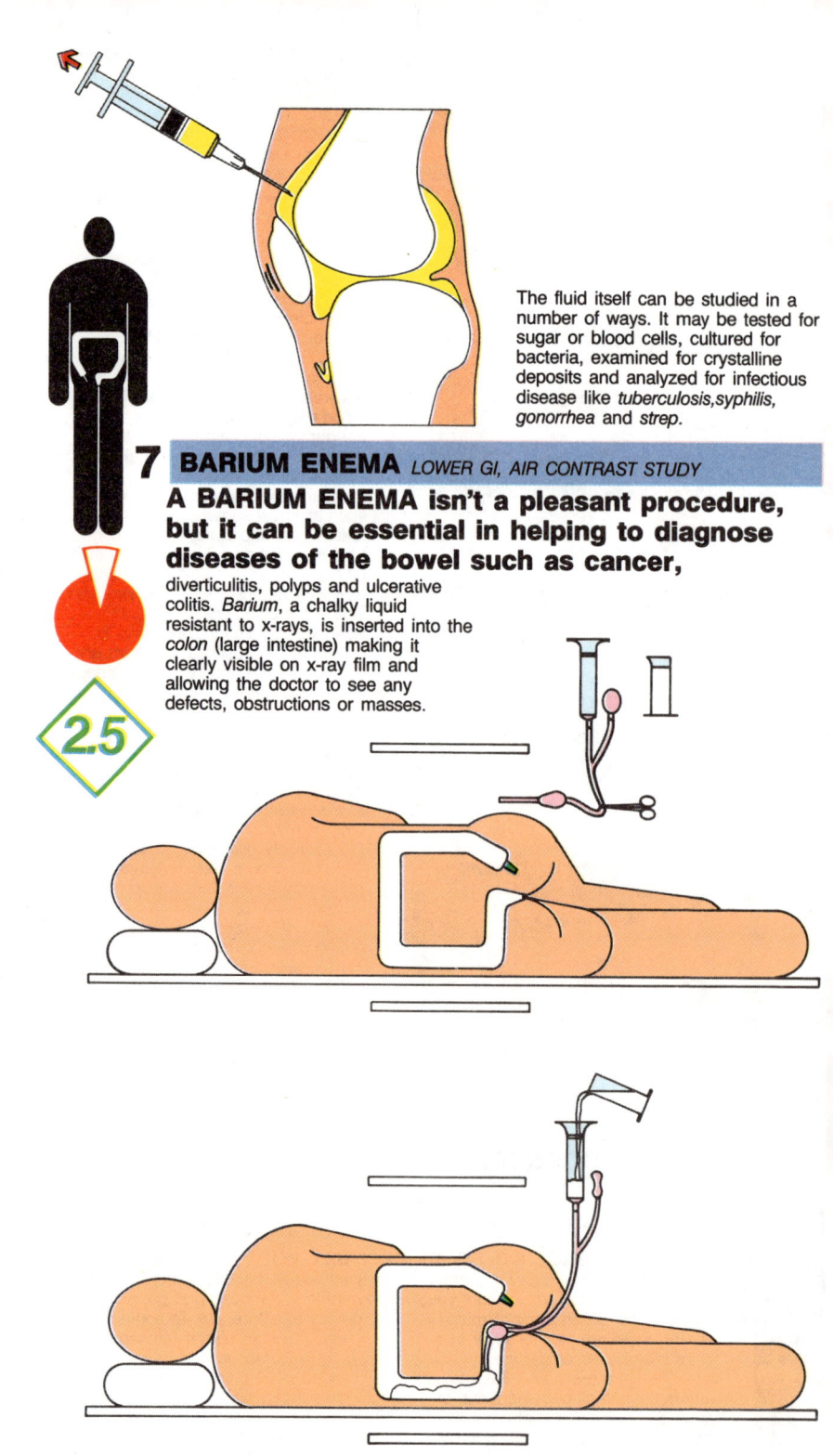

The fluid itself can be studied in a number of ways. It may be tested for sugar or blood cells, cultured for bacteria, examined for crystalline deposits and analyzed for infectious disease like *tuberculosis, syphilis, gonorrhea* and *strep*.

7 BARIUM ENEMA LOWER GI, AIR CONTRAST STUDY

A BARIUM ENEMA isn't a pleasant procedure, but it can be essential in helping to diagnose diseases of the bowel such as cancer, diverticulitis, polyps and ulcerative colitis. *Barium*, a chalky liquid resistant to x-rays, is inserted into the *colon* (large intestine) making it clearly visible on x-ray film and allowing the doctor to see any defects, obstructions or masses.

Since it is essential that the colon be clear of all gas and fecal matter, you will be instructed not to eat solids for 24 hours and not to drink for 8 hours before the test. You may be given laxatives and/or an enema the night before.

A regular abdominal x-ray is taken first. Then, you lie on your side while a lubricated nozzle is eased into your rectum. The barium fills the colon slowly, its progress often monitored on a fluoroscope (a TV that shows moving x-ray pictures). Pressure may be put on your abdomen to make sure the barium fills all the loops of the colon. Finally, several x-rays are taken.

With enemas it is usual to have a cramping feeling, fullness, and an overwhelming desire to defecate. A small balloon-type device on the tube helps you retain the barium. If you expel some of the liquid, don't be embarrassed. Doctors and technicians are used to it. Retaining your dignity and sense of humor can be as difficult as retaining the barium.

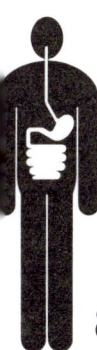

Once the x-rays are taken you are permitted to go to the bathroom and expel the barium, which will relieve much of your discomfort immediately. At this point—while the colon still has a light coating of barium—technicians may take more x-rays. Occasionally air is pumped into the colon for further x-rays. (This is particularly useful in diagnosing *polyps* or *small tumors.*) You may feel something like severe gas pains until you expel the forced air. A barium enema is not dangerous, just tiring, but it can be stressful for the very ill or old.

After the procedure you will probably be encouraged to drink lots of water to ease the constipation that often follows a barium enema—unless liquids are restricted for some other medical reason. Don't be alarmed if your stool is white for 24 to 72 hours. When a barium enema is part of a complete gastrointestinal series it is usually done first, before an **UPPER GI SERIES**.

8 BARIUM SWALLOW ESOPHOGRAM

This is generally considered the least tiring and uncomfortable of all the barium studies. The esophagus, the muscular tube that runs from the mouth to the top of the stomach, is usually given a quick check as part of an **UPPER GI**, but in some cases it is examined specifically. Problems related directly to the esophagus include *bleeding from ulcers* or *varicose veins, hiatal hernia, narrowing,* or *achalasia* (a difficulty in swallowing).

The test is done in the radiology department. You will probably be asked not to eat anything after midnight the night before. The technician stands you in front of a fluoroscopic unit with your back to an upright x-ray table. You are then given 4 ounces of thick chalky liquid to swallow. This is your *barium cocktail* or *barium milkshake,* which may be chocolate-, mint-, or banana-flavored. (The flavorings and the cute names do little to make the barium palatable. The stuff tastes terrible, no matter what.) As you swallow, the radiologist stands in a booth and watches a video of the barium going down the esophagus. Spot x-rays are taken, and sometimes the whole thing is recorded on videotape.

In some cases you lie on a table with your head slightly lower than your feet while the x-rays are taken. This allows the radiologist to follow the barium at a slower pace. If you have had spasms in the esophagus, you may be given a piece of bread soaked in barium to swallow. That way the radiologist can see what typically happens when food is swallowed.

The whole process should be over in 15 to 30 minutes and there should be no ill effects afterwards except for possible constipation. Drinking lots of fluids will ease this. Your stool will probably be white for at least 24 hours.

9 BILIRUBIN

The average life span of a red blood cell is four months. As it dies it gives off hemoglobin. The hemoglobin is carried by the bloodstream to the liver, where it is broken down into bilirubin, a golden-colored waste product that can be easily eliminated. Bilirubin flows from the liver to the gallbladder in bile, and from there to the intestines. Finally it is eliminated by the bowel, imparting the characteristic dark color to feces.

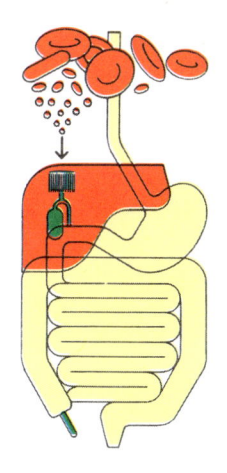

Typically, only small amounts of the chemical are present in the blood. When the level is elevated, it means less than the normal amount of bilirubin is being processed and excreted. (High levels may also be present in certain *anemias* when red blood cells are dying at an abnormally high rate.) Patients with excess bilirubin will often have the yellowish tinge to skin and eyes associated with jaundice

Testing for bilirubin is common when *liver disease,* or *obstruction of the bile ducts by gallstones* or *pancreatic cancer* is suspected. Though the test is considered a highly accurate indicator of liver disease, it is not helpful in distinguishing among the many varieties. Therefore, it is often ordered in conjunction with several other **Liver Function Tests.**

In order for your physician to make the correct interpretation of results, he or she must know if you are taking *medication.* Thorazine, male hormones, certain antibiotics and arthritis pain medicine can increase bilirubin levels, as can fasting and dieting. The test itself is a simple blood test and is frequently part of a multiple test panel.

Urine usually contains no bilirubin; however, it too may be tested when liver disease or obstruction of the bile ducts is suspected.

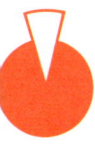

10 BLOOD PRESSURE

Over 37 million Americans have high blood pressure. In most cases there are no warning symptoms, so for many, the first time they find out about the problem is a surprise. High blood pressure is implicated as a major factor in deaths from heart attack, heart failure and stroke—that's over a million funerals a year. On the plus side, high blood pressure is easily detected by a simple, painless test, and once detected, can be controlled very effectively.

Everyone has blood pressure. It is the pressure or tension of the blood against the artery walls, as it is forced by the heart through the body. Though this pressure fluctuates with every heart beat—highest when the heart contracts, lowest when it relaxes—and responds to changes in your activity (it almost doubles during sex), it is always there. In cases of high blood pressure, also called *hypertension*, the heart encounters resistance and must work harder to pump the blood.

Over time, the heart enlarges. A slight enlargement may pose no problem, but at a certain point, an enlarged heart grows weaker and is unable to function. High blood pressure also increases wear and tear on the arteries. Some may weaken to the point of bursting, which in the brain could cause a stroke. It also seems that arteries damaged by high blood pressure are more likely to develop buildups of fatty *plaques*. They become narrower, less elastic and may be unable to deliver all the blood that is needed by the body. Again, the heart is forced to work harder. People with high blood pressure are also more likely to form blood clots, which may get trapped in a narrow blood vessel and deprive a part of the body of needed blood.

Blood pressure readings are given as 2 numbers: 120/80 (read, *120 over 80*), for example. The top number, *the systolic pressure,* refers to the pressure in your arteries right after the heart has contracted, when the force is highest. The bottom number, *diastolic pressure,* is a measurement of the pressure in your arteries when the heart is momentarily relaxing between beats. The measurement is taken with a *sphygmomanometer,* a machine that measures your blood pressure by comparing the pressure inside the major artery in your arm with air pressure inside an inflatable cuff. While there are new electronic machines that measure blood pressure, most doctors still use the conventional equipment, which includes a stethoscope and an inflatable arm cuff that is attached to a mercury-filled pressure gauge or a dial.

The test is usually performed in a doctor's office while you are lying or sitting down. The examiner wraps the cuff around your upper arm and places the stethoscope over the main artery in the inside of your elbow. (This is one of several points, including your neck and the inside of your wrist, where you should be able to feel your own pulse.)

It is hard to establish what exactly is normal blood pressure. Though 120/80 has traditionally been given as the normal figure, it's rare that anyone comes in with a reading that's right on the mark. In general, high levels in the diastolic, or bottom number, are thought to be more important than high levels in the upper number. Anyone with a diastolic pressure of 85 or less is considered in good shape. Diastolic pressure between 85 and 89 warrants a follow-up exam within the year. 90 to 114 is considered moderate hypertension and may require treatment. Above that, the hypertension is severe and demands immediate attention.

The examiner inflates the cuff until external pressure is greater than the pressure inside the artery. The artery momentarily collapses and circulation stops. Then, as the examiner slowly lowers the cuff pressure by releasing air through a valve, she listens through the stethoscope. Soon she hears a thumping sound as blood is forced through the artery in spurts. She looks at the pressure gauge and notes the number. This is the *systolic pressure* or maximum blood pressure. More air is released from the cuff, the thumps become lighter. When pressure outside the artery is equal to pressure inside the artery and no thumps at all can be heard, the gauge is read again. This number is the *diastolic* or minimum blood pressure.

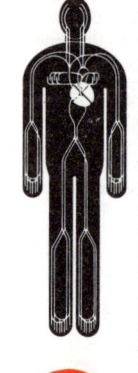

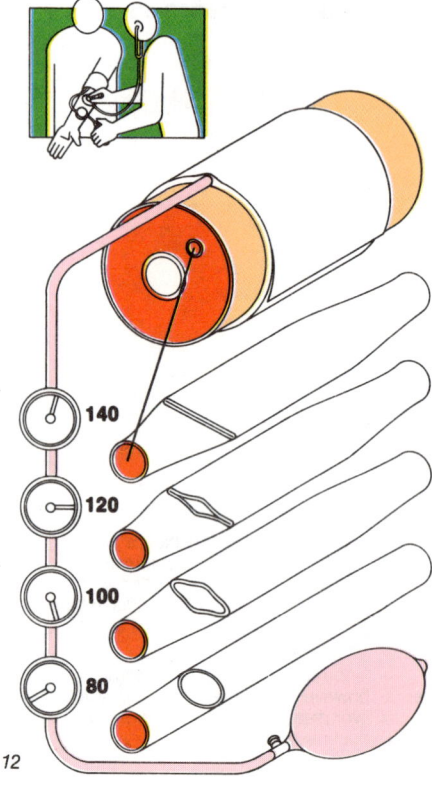

The results of a blood pressure reading depend on a number of factors: the force of the heart beat, the elasticity of the arterial walls, the volume of blood, the thickness of the blood and amount of dissolved chemicals in it, hormone levels, and drugs like birth control pills. Your posture and reactions to stress can affect your blood pressure as well. Sometimes, just being in the doctor's office can make you nervous enough to raise your blood pressure. For that reason, many doctors like to take blood pressure readings once at the beginning of an exam, and again towards the end, when the patient has, one hopes, relaxed. In any event, a diagnosis of high blood pressure cannot be based on 1 reading though 1 high reading should serve as notice to check again. Ideally, a diagnosis is made after several readings have been taken over a period of time.

Your doctor may refer to 2 kinds of hypertension: *essential* and *secondary*. Secondary hypertension is caused by a specific problem like kidney disease, diabetes, or thyroid gland malfunction. In many cases, when the underlying problem is treated, the high blood pressure goes away. However, at least 90 percent of those with high blood pressure have essential hypertension. No one knows exactly what causes essential hypertension. There is, however, a lot of information about what makes it worse. Being overweight, eating a high salt diet and extreme tension all contribute to the problem. In many cases, eliminating these irritating factors by changes in lifestyle is all that is needed to control the condition. If that is not sufficient, there are a number of drugs that can help. In most cases, you will have to take the drugs for life; on the other hand, the life may be a lot longer.

The importance of having your blood pressure tested regularly cannot be overstressed. Though some people do experience symptoms of hypertension like *headaches, palpitations*, and a *general feeling of ill health*, these symptoms do not appear until the condition is already very dangerous. The most common symptom of severe hypertension is sudden death. It is almost universally recommended that adults have their blood pressure checked at least every other year, more frequently if there is a family history of hypertension.

BLOOD TESTS

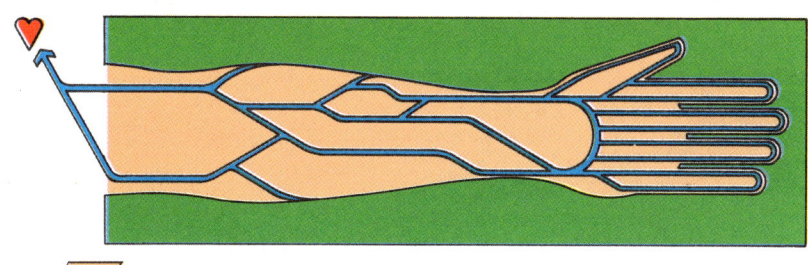

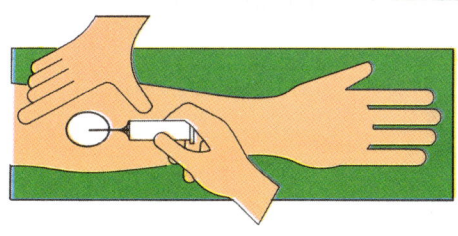

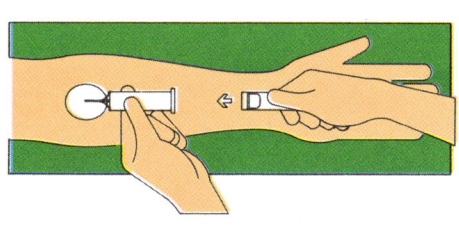

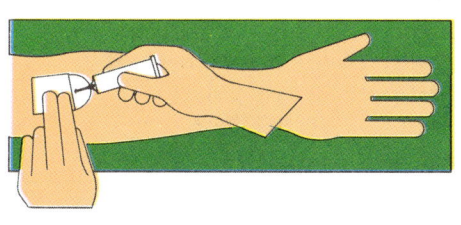

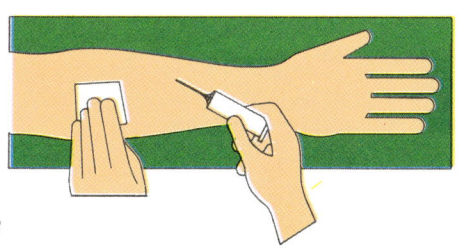

Venipuncture is the method with which most of us are familiar. A tourniquet is wrapped around the upper arm. This blocks the flow of blood in the veins and makes them stand out a bit more. The technician then feels for a vein and cleans the area with an alcohol swab. (The *median cephalic vein,* which is inside the crook of your arm and slightly to the right, is the vein of choice but any of several others can be used.) A needle connection to either a syringe or a glass vacuum tube is quickly inserted in the vein. If a syringe is used, the technician pulls back gently on the plunger. If a vacuum tube is used, the blood simply flows into it. After the sample is obtained, a cotton ball is put on and pressure is applied to the site of the needle prick. Later a bandaid is put on in its place.

In the hands of a skilled technician, this should be quick and not very painful. There is no risk to speak of from a blood test; though patients, particularly older patients whose veins are difficult to locate, may be stuck several times. This can cause a bruise which may take a week or so to clear up. The amount of blood withdrawn is not enough to make a patient weak, but people have been known to get dizzy and faint just at the sight of it. This is awkward, but not dangerous, since you are always lying down or seated in a chair when blood is drawn.

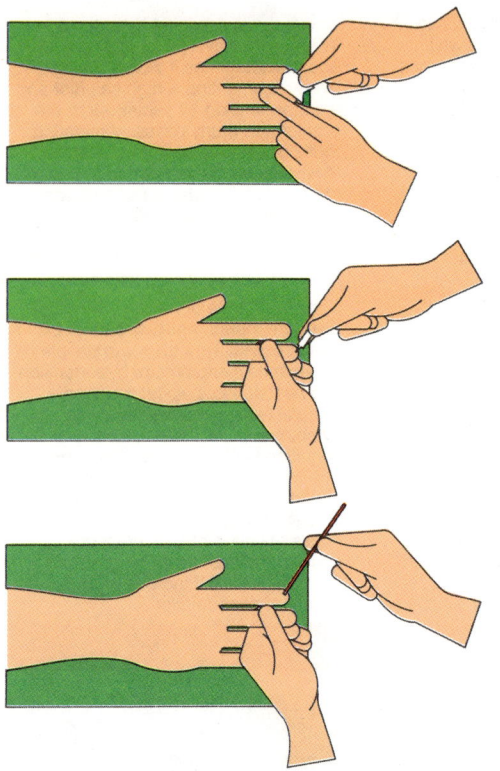

hurts just about as much and the finger may be sore for a day or two. If you are in the hospital, you may be awakened for blood testing very early in the morning. Certainly this is not the kind of treatment you want in a room that may cost a hundred dollars a day, but the levels of many chemicals in the blood fluctuate. Often the truest reading is obtained first thing in the morning, before you have had breakfast. You may also find that your blood is tested every day or several times during the day. This may be necessary to monitor drug dosage or the course of infection, and though it is annoying, it is not dangerous. A full series of blood tests require about an ounce of blood—less than 1 percent of the total, and easily replaceable in a day.

When your doctor orders a particular blood test, or perhaps wants to get a general overview of your health, he may order something called an **SMA 6, SMA 12** or **SMA 24. SMA** stands for sequential multiple analyzer, a machine that can run a series of chemical tests on 1 blood sample at the same time. This test may also be referred to as a multiple test panel, chemistry panel or blood profile. SMAs don't cost any more than regular blood tests; in fact some labs automatically perform them even when only one specific test on the panel is requested. The extra information may help your doctor get an overall look at many interrelated systems. On the other hand, when so many tests are performed at once, the odds increase that at least one of the test results will be wrong. Estimates put the chance of a healthy person having at least one false positive in a 12-part test at roughly 30 percent. Obviously no important diagnosis should be made just on the basis of an SMA.

The **fingerstick method.** It is usually employed on children, patients who are scared of *venipuncture,* and often in blood donation centers where only a little bit of blood is needed to do the basic screening tests. It may also be used if your doctor is using some of the newer automated machines to perform a Complete Blood Count in his office.

Your finger is cleaned with an alcohol swab, and grasped firmly. Then the tip is quickly jabbed with a sharp sterile piece of metal called a *lancet.* The technician gently squeezes the finger until blood flows. Blood is drawn up in a *pipette,* a very thin glass tube which is touched to the finger. In a variation of this method, called the *heelstick,* the bottom of the foot is pierced. This method is used almost exclusively on newborn babies whose blood is routinely screened after birth. Many think the fingerstick method is less painful than a vein stick. In fact, it

The body must produce 2,400,000 red cells per second in order to maintain a normal concentration of blood.

The total surface area of the red cells, in an average person, is 3820 square meters, about 2000 times greater than his or her total body surface area.

The average person has approximately 10½ pints of blood in circulation, which constitutes about 7-8 percent of the body weight.

11 COMPLETE BLOOD COUNT CBC

A Complete Blood Count (CBC) is performed more frequently than any other blood test. It is often included in a complete physical and is

performed as a matter of course on almost all patients entering the hospital. The most common reasons for performing the test are to screen for *anemia* (too few red cells) or *infection* (too many white cells). But the test also provides the physician with a tremendous amount of information on overall health and the health of the blood manufacturing mechanism in particular.

A complete blood count is actually a collection of several individual tests usually performed at the same time by a *Coulter Counter,* a machine that automatically separates blood into its individual components and measures them. Generally all the individual tests are ordered together, in which case one small sample of blood (about 2-3 teaspoons) is drawn from a vein in the arm. However, when only a few of the individual tests are needed, the sample may be taken by the fingerstick method, in which only a few drops are drawn up a thin glass tube.

A complete blood count usually contains the following tests:

Red blood cell count. Red blood cells (erythrocytes) are the most common type of blood cell. (The average person has about 35 trillion of them.) They are responsible for transporting oxygen throughout the body and bringing waste carbon dioxide back to the lungs where it can be expelled.

In this test, the amount of cells in 1 cubic millimeter of blood is calculated and compared to a list of normal values depending on age, sex and, in some cases, altitude. (People who live in mountainous areas typically have more red blood cells than those living at sea level. This environmental adaptation helps compensate for the reduced oxygen at high altitudes.)

Low levels are associated with *anemias, severe infections, iron* and *vitamin B12 deficiencies, malarias, prolonged internal bleeding* and certain types of *cancer*.

Red blood cells may also be stained and examined under a microscope for their size, shape and maturity. This part of the test, which may be called a *red cell differential* or *peripheral blood smear,* can help further diagnose anemias and identify malaria.

Hemoglobin is the main component of red blood cells and has the all-important chemical attraction to oxygen. In general, hemoglobin levels are closely linked to the red blood cell count. Certain iron deficiency anemias, however, can cause a lower hemoglobin level, while the red blood cell level remains close to normal. Hemoglobin levels also tend to reflect overall blood volume. Hemoglobin levels are high, for instance, in cases of dehydration.

Hematocrit. Blood is made up of white cells, red cells, platelets and about 78 percent plasma, a watery solution of dissolved proteins and minerals. A hematocrit measures how much of the total blood volume is made up of red blood cells. Abnormal values indicate basically the same conditions as do abnormal red blood cell and hemoglobin tests, but there are subtle differences that can be used to differentiate among types of anemia. A potential blood donor is usually given a hematocrit (by the finger prick method) to determine if his or her red blood volume is sufficient for safe donation.

White blood cell count and differential. There is 1 white blood cell for every 1000 red blood cells, but that proportion does not reflect their importance. The white cells are responsible for fighting infection; the body typically responds to bacterial or foreign invasion by producing more of them. A white blood cell count, therefore, is an important part of any investigation of infection. It may be ordered when you present symptoms of *fever* or *swollen glands*. It is also commonly performed after surgery to make sure no infection has developed. Stress and trauma may also raise your white blood cell count. Massive infections, drug or poison reactions, and chemotherapy may lower it.

There are actually 5 different types of white blood cells; some directly attack bacteria, while others produce antibodies to fight it. Some are more common in the early stages of infection, and some in later stages. A *differential* is the part of the test in which relative percentages of the various white cells are calculated. An increase in any 1 type of cell can help indicate the type of infection involved and the effectiveness with which the body is combatting it. For this part of the test, a drop of blood is smeared on a slide, stained and then examined, either mechanically or under a microscope by a trained examiner or *hematologist,* a doctor specializing in diseases of the blood. (A white blood cell differential and red blood cell differential are sometimes done at the same time as a test called *peripheral blood smear.*)

Platelet count. Sometimes included in a CBC, this test measures the amount of platelets in a cubic millimeter of blood. Platelets are not actually cells, but rather cell fragments that play an essential part in clot formation—a deficiency may lead to dangerous internal bleeding. Platelet count can be affected by a variety of conditions, including extreme blood loss or tissue injury, *anemias, leukemia* and certain cancers. This test may be done with other tests of the blood's clotting mechanism before surgery or a tooth extraction.

12 ACID PHOSPHATASE

Measures the blood level of an enzyme that is concentrated in the prostate gland. High levels of acid phosphatase are released into the blood when there is *prostate cancer*. The test may be used as a basic screening test for older men, but it's more commonly used to monitor the effectiveness of treatment in men who already have a diagnosis for prostate cancer. False positive results may occur if the prostate has been examined manually preceding the acid phosphatase blood test. The test should not be conducted on a day when you have a rectal exam.

13 AIDS ACQUIRED IMMUNE DEFICIENCY SYNDROME

There is no blood test to diagnose AIDS. However, there is a test, licensed by the government in March of 1985, that screens the blood for antibodies, which are produced by the body in response to the virus suspected of causing AIDS. The test does not show whether someone who tests positive has AIDS or will ever get it. Antibodies (the immune system's response to invasion) in the blood merely indicate that someone was once exposed to the virus. It is more than likely that the exposed person's immune system has effectively fended off the virus. Current studies by the Centers for Disease Control in Atlanta indicate that only 1-2 percent of all people who test positive will ever contract the disease. (See **2**)

14 ALCOHOL

Measures the blood level of alcohol, normally not found in the body at all. When evaluating a potential drunk driver, police are likely to use a breath test. In many states, however, those accused can demand a blood test. In most states a blood alcohol level between 0.1 and 0.5 percent is considered legal proof of intoxication—however, anything over 0.05 percent significantly impairs driving ability. In a hospital, blood alcohol may be tested whenever a patient is brought into the emergency room in a coma or behaving abnormally. It is important when taking the blood sample to clean the arm with something other than alcohol. (See **3**)

15 ALKALINE PHOSPHATASE

Measures the blood level of an enzyme found in both bone and liver. When disease causes destruction of liver cells the enzyme seeps into the blood. Levels may be high in cases of liver cancer or *inflammation, hepatitis,* and *bile duct obstruction* by gallstones. Male hormones, birth control pills and some tranquilizers and antibiotics can also cause elevated levels. Alkaline phosphatase is also raised in *bone disease* and when bone *fractures* are healing. Alkaline phosphatase is always included in a series of **LIVER FUNCTION TESTS** and often in a multiple test panel.

16 ALPHAFETOPROTEIN *AFP*

Measures the blood level of alphafetoprotein which can be elevated in *cancer of the liver, cancer of the testicles* and in some instances of *hepatitis.* If it remains elevated following removal of a testicular cancer, it means that there is still residual cancer elsewhere in the body. Amniotic fluid is also tested for AFP, where abnormal levels may indicate birth defects such as *spina bifida.* (For further information see **AMNIOCENTESIS**.)

17 AMYLASE

Measures the blood level of an enzyme produced by the pancreas and essential in the digestion of starches. High blood levels may indicate pancreatic disease such as *pancreatitis, cancer* or *cystic disease of the pancreas.* Amylase is usually tested with **LIPASE**, another pancreatic enzyme. Urine is also tested for amylase and lipase.

18 BILIRUBIN

Measures the blood level of bilirubin, the end product of the natural breakdown of red blood cells. The test is performed when there is a suspicion of *liver disease, bile duct obstruction* and certain *anemias* (blood diseases). The test is included in a multiple screening panel and in **LIVER FUNCTION TESTS**. Any patient with signs of jaundice (yellowing of the skin and the whites of the eyes) will be tested for bilirubin. (See **9**)

19 BLOOD TYPING & CROSS MATCH

Determines which of the 4 main blood groups, A, B, AB, or O your blood belongs to. It is essential before transfusion and is always done as part of a pre-surgery workup. Cross matching helps identify any other incompatibilities that might exist between the donor's and recipient's blood.

20 BLOOD UREA NITROGEN *BUN*

Measures the blood level of urea nitrogen, a waste chemical that is normally filtered out of the blood by the kidneys. This is probably the most common screening test for kidney function and is almost always included in a multiple test panel. It may also be used to assess the severity of dehydration.

21 CALCIUM

Measures the blood level of calcium, a mineral stored in the bones and essential for a variety of functions, including heart muscle contraction and nerve impulse transmission. Calcium levels are regulated by the Parathyroid gland. High levels may indicate *parathyroid malfunction, myeloma,* a type of bone cancer (most common in men over 40) or other *cancers* which have spread to the bone. Low calcium levels are found in people with *kidney disease* or *vitamin D deficiency*. This is a general screening test often performed with Magnesium and **PHOSPHORUS** in a multiple test panel.

22 CARCINOEMBRYONIC ANTIGEN *CEA*

Measures blood level of CEA, a chemical which is frequently elevated in cases of *bowel, rectal, lung, stomach* and *breast cancer.* It is not specific enough to be a diagnostic test, but is frequently used to monitor the effectiveness of treatment on patients who have already been diagnosed for cancer, especially bowel cancer. Smokers may have slightly elevated levels of CEA.

23 CHOLESTEROL

Measures the amount of cholesterol circulating in the blood. Cholesterol is manufactured by the body itself, as well as being found in animal foodstuffs like meat, eggs and milk. It is a structural part of every cell, aids in hormone production and is essential to brain and nerve development. Although high amounts of cholesterol have been linked to *fatty deposits* in the arteries and a higher risk of *heart attack,* the exact causal connection between cholesterol and heart disease is still the object of medical debate. Cholesterol may be tested when screening for risk of *heart disease* or when assessing the effectiveness of diet and exercise in lowering previously diagnosed high levels. Cholesterol combines with triglycerides in the blood to form complex molecules called *Lipoproteins* which must also be measured when assessing for risk of heart disease. Cholesterol is measured in milligrams per 100 milliliters of blood. Normal levels have not been satisfactorily determined. But anything over 300 is cause for concern. (See **90**)

24 COOMBS' TEST

Analyzes the blood for the presence of antibodies directed toward the patient's own red blood cells. Used when matching blood for transfusion and diagnosing certain anemias and diseases of the immune system.

25 CREATINE PHOSPHOKINASE *CPK, CK*

Measures the blood level of Creatine Phosphokinase, an enzyme found in heart muscle, skeletal muscle (e.g., arm, leg) and the brain. Damage to any of the above can elevate the blood level. Most frequently used to diagnose or monitor *heart attack* patients and patients with chest pains. May also be used in diagnosing *muscular dystrophy*. (See **CARDIAC ENZYMES**.)

26 CREATININE

Measures the blood level of Creatinine, a waste product that is filtered out of the blood by the kidneys. Higher than usual levels of this substance may indicate *kidney disease*. This is a common test of kidney function and is often included in a multiple test panel. (See **CREATININE CLEARANCE**.)

27 ERYTHROCYTE SEDIMENTATION RATE *SED RATE, ESR*

A screening test used to evaluate overall health. A blood sample is taken and observed later to determine what percentage of red blood cells has settled to the bottom of a test tube after 1 hour has elapsed. Where there is *inflammation, arthritis, infection* or *cancer*, the red blood cells settle faster. Often used to check on the recovery of patients with infectious disease. The SED rate is also elevated in *pregnancy*. This test is often performed in the doctor's office.

28 FASTING BLOOD SUGAR

Similar to glucose or blood sugar test, except the patient is asked not to eat for 8 hours before the test. This is one of the major tests used to diagnose diabetes. It may be used alone or in conjunction with other blood tests that measure the body's reaction to glucose.

29 GASTRIN

Measures the blood level of a hormone that stimulates intestinal movement and the secretion of digestive juices. May be ordered to evaluate severe and chronic peptic ulcer disease. (In *Zollinger-Ellison Syndrome* gastrin producing tumors provoke multiple *peptic ulcers*.)

30 GLUCOSE *BLOOD SUGAR*

Measures the amount of glucose (sugar) in the blood. A glucose test is always part of a multiple test panel because it's a good screening test for several metabolic diseases, most notably *diabetes*, where glucose is high, and *hypoglycemia*, where glucose is low. Thyroid and adrenal gland disease may affect glucose levels as can *diuretics* (water pills). This test is performed frequently on newly diagnosed diabetics while determining the correct insulin dose. Urine may also be tested.

31 GLUCOSE TOLERANCE TEST *GTT*

Measures very precisely the body's ability to process sugar, and is a commonly used test in diagnosis of *diabetes* and *hypoglycemia*. You must eat a high starch diet for 3 days, then fast from midnight until the morning of the test. Blood and urine samples are taken before you are given a measured amount of glucose (usually a highly sugared drink). Blood samples are taken 5 to 6 times over the next 5 hours and analyzed for sugar levels. You will have to remain in the lab, doctor's office or hospital for the duration of the test.

32 HEPATITIS

There are several related blood tests used to determine if a patient has been exposed to viral hepatitis, is currently infected with the virus, or is no longer infected but is still a carrier. Tests also differentiate between Hepatitis A (*infectious hepatitis*), which is fairly mild and Hepatitis B (*serum hepatitis*), a much more severe disease that may require hospitalization. The most common test is called the Hepatitis B surface Antigen test (HBsAg) which detects the virus in the blood and measures its strength. (See **83**)

33 IRON & TOTAL IRON BINDING CAPACITY *TIBC*

These 2 tests, almost always done together, measure the amount of iron in the blood. Iron is essential for the production of hemoglobin and healthy red blood cells. The test is ordered when *iron deficiency anemia* is suspected. Possible causes are dietary deficiency, lack of absorption in the intestines and blood loss, either in the digestive tract or through excessive menstrual bleeding. Often included in a multiple test panel.

34 KETONES

Measures ketone levels in blood. Ketones are chemical compounds produced when the body is unable to use carbohydrates and is forced to burn fat reserves. The test may be performed when assessing *diabetes*, the effects of *starvation*, or *dehydration* due to vomiting or diarrhea. Blood and urine are tested.

35 LACTIC DEHYDROGENASE *LDH*

Measures the blood level of Lactic Dehydrogenase, an enzyme present in heart muscle, liver, lung and kidney tissue, and released into the blood when one of the above has been damaged. Used primarily in diagnosis of *heart attack* and *liver disease*. LDH is also elevated in cases of advanced *cancer*. If you're hospitalized for heart attack or undiagnosed chest pains, the test may be performed every day. (See **63** & **92**.)

36 LEAD

Measures the amount of lead in the blood. Only very low amounts should be present. High levels may indicate lead poisoning. Symptoms of lead poisoning include *diarrhea, abdominal pain* and *behavioral changes*. Those most at risk are children who eat paint chips or chew on old painted toys and furniture. This is a common screening test for young children.

37 LIPASE

Measures the blood level of an enzyme produced by the pancreas and used in the digestion of fats. High levels are present in *pancreatitis* (inflammation of the pancreas) and *cysts*. Perhaps a bit less sensitive than the **AMYLASE** test, but useful because when there is pancreatic disease the lipase level will remain high for several days after the amylase has returned to normal. Lipase may also be measured in the urine.

38 LIPIDS *LIPOPROTEINS*

Measures the blood level of fats like cholesterol and triglycerides. Used mainly as an indicator of risk for *coronary artery disease*. Once in the blood, these fats join with proteins to form complex molecules called lipoproteins, two of which, HDLs (high-density lipoproteins) and LDLs (low-density lipoproteins) are particularly significant for heart disease. LDLs seem to increase risk while HDLs seem to lower it. A full lipid or blood fat analysis includes total cholesterol and triglyceride levels and a lipoprotein profile. (See **90**)

39 MONONUCLEOSIS *MONO–SPOT*

Detects the presence of antibodies in the blood that fight the mononucleosis virus. The most common test is called the **Mono–Spot Test** and can be performed in a doctor's office. Anyone, particularly a youngster, who presents the symptoms—*headache, sore throat, swollen glands, abdominal pain, fever, malaise*—may be given this screening test. If the results are positive another blood test, the Heterophile Test, is needed to confirm the diagnosis. This test must be sent to a lab for analysis.

40 OSMOLALITY

A measure of the *thickness* of the blood, the concentration of solids, salts, sugars, fats and other chemicals. Despite extreme variations in dietary intake the body manages to keep osmolality at a fairly constant level. However, any radical disturbance of water balance will affect osmolality. This might be true in cases of extreme *vomiting, diarrhea, diabetes malitus, diabetes insipidus, kidney* and *brain disease*. The test is not specific for any one disease, but because the body's water balance is intimately connected with the health of many organs and metabolic processes, it's often included in a comprehensive multiple screening panel. Urine may also be tested for osmolality.

41 PARTIAL THROMBOPLASTIN TIME *PTT*

There are over a dozen chemicals, or *factors*, that control how fast your blood clots. The PTT Test can detect abnormally low levels in 8 of them. Because it is a measure of clotting time, the test is often part of pre-surgery workup. Also used when monitoring patients on blood thinning medication like *heparin* and when diagnosing clotting diseases like *hemophilia*. (Hemophilia is associated with low levels of Factor VIII or IX.)

42 PHOSPHORUS

Measures the blood level of phosphorus, a chemical that's involved in a number of body functions including bone formation and carbohydrate metabolism. Abnormal levels are found where there is *kidney disease, malfunctioning parathyroid glands* or abnormally *high* or *low vitamin D* levels. Not strictly diagnostic of anything, but useful in giving your doctor an overall view of your health. Often included in the larger multiple test panels.

43 PHENYLKETONURIA *PKU, GUTHRIE TEST*

A test performed on all newborn infants to identify a genetic disorder in which the child can't metabolize a chemical (phenylalinine) needed for normal growth. Untreated, the disorder causes *mental retardation*, but if detected early, and treated with a special diet, normal development is practically assured.

44 POTASSIUM

Tests the blood level of potassium, a mineral involved in a variety of essential functions including muscle contraction, nerve impulse conduction and maintenance of the body's acid-base and water balances. In most cases an insufficiency is not related to diet, but rather to *diuretic* drugs used to treat high blood pressure–they cause an excessive loss of the mineral in urine. A severe imbalance in the potassium level can bring on *muscle weakness* and possibly life-threatening *irregular heart rhythms*. This test, while not in itself diagnostic for any specific disease, is useful in getting an overview of your metabolism. Patients with *heart* or *kidney disease, high blood pressure* (especially those on *diuretics*), or *diabetes* are apt to be tested more frequently than others. The test is included in an **electrolyte** panel and most multiple test panels. (See **76**)

45 PROTEIN, ALBUMIN GLOBULIN RATIO *A/G RATIO*

These 2 tests measure the levels of albumin and globulin, the 2 main proteins in the blood. They provide nourishment for muscle and organ tissue as well as transporting vitamins, enzymes, hormones and disease fighting agents throughout the body. A typical multiple test panel will measure the total amount of blood protein as well as the ratio of albumin to globulin. Abnormal levels or altered ratios are seen in a wide variety of conditions including *liver* and *kidney disease, dehydration, chronic infection* and certain types of *cancer*. These are screening tests used to narrow the diagnostic field or help confirm a diagnosis. They are not in themselves diagnostic.

46. PROTHROMBIN TIME *PT, PRO TIME*

Measures how quickly the chemicals that control blood clotting work. Often part of a pre-surgery group of screening tests. Also used in diagnosing *liver disease* and monitoring patients on oral blood thinning medication.

47. RHEUMATOID FACTOR

Tests the blood for presence of the rheumatoid factor, an antibody present in *rheumatoid arthritis,* an inflammatory disease of the joints.

48. RUBELLA TITER *GERMAN MEASLES*

Tests the blood for the presence of antibodies that fight against German measles. German measles is a fairly mild disease common in school age children. However, if it's contracted by a pregnant woman, particularly in the first trimester, there is a 50 percent chance the infant will be born with severe birth defects. Presence of rubella antibody in the blood shows that the person tested was once exposed to the disease and is now immune. If no antibody is present, the patient should be vaccinated. California, Colorado, New Jersey and Rhode Island require women to be tested before they can receive a marriage license. All 50 states require children to be vaccinated. A rubella titer is a common screening test for teenage girls, women contemplating pregnancy and women who are already pregnant.

49. SGOT *SERUM GLUTAMIC OXALOACETIC TRANSAMINASE*

Measures the blood level of an enzyme found primarily in heart and liver tissue. Damage to the heart or liver results in higher blood levels. SGOT is released into the blood 24-48 hours after a *heart attack* and remains in the blood for 5 days. Usually performed in conjunction with other heart or liver tests. (See **63** & **91**)

50. SGPT *SERUM GLUTAMIC PYRUVIC TRANSAMINASE*

Measures the blood level of an enzyme found primarily in the liver. High levels in the blood indicate an injured or diseased liver. A common liver function test. (See **92**)

51. SICKLE CELL ANEMIA *SICKLADEX*

Sickle cell anemia is a genetically transmitted blood disease, found primarily, but not exclusively, among blacks. The main ingredient of a healthy red blood cell is *hemoglobin A.* The red blood cells of a person with sickle cell disease are made up almost entirely of an abnormal hemoglobin, *hemoglobin S.* These cells are fragile and die easily which often results in anemia. When the level of oxygen in the blood falls even slightly, the hemoglobin S cells change their shape and become crescent or sickle-shaped. The sickled cells can form *plugs* or *clots* in the small blood vessels of various organs, causing acute attacks of pain and in some instances tissue death.

Persons with only one sickle cell gene are said to have the sickle cell trait. (There is some small amount of the abnormal hemoglobin in their blood, but not enough to cause any ill effects.) There are several blood tests designed to detect sickle cell anemia and sickle cell trait. In the most common screening test, a small blood sample is taken, oxygen is removed from the blood and the sample is examined for signs of sickling. To make a more precise diagnosis, *hemoglobin electrophoreisis* is performed. In this test, a blood sample is electrically charged which causes the different varieties of hemoglobin to separate.

52. SODIUM

Measures the blood level of sodium (salt), one of the main mineral components of blood. Sodium maintains the body's internal water balance and is essential for proper muscle contraction and nerve impulse conduction. Though dietary intake may vary from 2 to 12 grams a day, the kidney and the brain work together to maintain the salt level within very narrow limits. Fluctuations are seen in *fever, dehydration* due to diarrhea, *vomiting,* and extreme *heat exposure.* Hormone disorders, *kidney* and *heart disease* and *high blood pressure* are all affected by and in turn act on the blood sodium level. The test is often ordered to monitor patients whose high blood pressure is being treated with *diuretics.* Sodium is often included in a multiple test panel or in an electrolyte panel.(See **76**)

53. SYPHILIS *VDRL, FTA-ABS*

Analyzes the blood for the presence of antibodies produced in response to the microorganism that causes syphilis. Probably the most common screening test is a VDRL (Venereal Disease Research Lab). If the results are positive, they must be confirmed with the FTA-ABS test, which is more specific and slightly more expensive. Anyone with syphilis should be tested again after treatment. Anyone with gonorrhea should also be tested for syphilis as a matter of course. (See **110**)

54. TAY SACHS

Tay Sachs is an inherited disease of the metabolism found primarily, but not exclusively, among Ashkenazic Jews, i.e., Jews of Eastern European descent. Tay Sachs victims are missing *hexosaminidase A,* an essential enzyme. Without it, a fat compound accumulates in the cells of the nervous system. Tay Sachs babies are born healthy, but begin to show signs of nervous system damage within 4 months. This is followed by blindness, seizures and inevitably by death between the ages of 3 and 5. Approximately 1 in 30 Ashkenazic Jews is a carrier and 1 out of every 25,000 Ashkenazic newborns will have the disease. Carriers have no symptoms and lead normal lives. Carriers are easily identified by analyzing a blood sample (which will have lower than average but safe levels of the enzyme). Testing is strongly recommended when both members of a couple are Ashkenazic Jews. A couple where both parents are carriers has a 25 percent chance of producing a Tay Sachs baby. Tay Sachs can be detected in a fetus through **AMNIOCENTESIS**. Some couples consider therapeutic abortion.

55 THYROXINE

Measures the amount of one of several thyroid hormones circulating in the blood, and is an accurate gauge of thyroid gland function. High levels indicate *hyperthyroidism*. Symptoms may include *sweatiness, increased heart rate, nervousness, diarrhea, weight loss and a feeling of being hot*. Low levels indicate *hypothyroidism*. Symptoms are *constipation, weight gain, fatigue and sensitivity to cold*. Other tests are usually required to determine the cause of the imbalance. (See **THYROID FUNCTION TESTS**.)

56 THYROID STIMULATING HORMONE *TSH*

Measures the blood level of TSH, a hormone produced at the base of the brain by the pituitary gland. When thyroid hormone levels are too high the TSH level decreases which signals the thyroid gland to cut back production. When thyroid hormone levels are too low, TSH secretion increases and acts as a signal to the thyroid gland to produce more hormone. The test is often one of a group of tests used to analyze thyroid function. Its chief use is in distinguishing between *hypothyroidism* (underactive thyroid gland) caused by a malfunction of the thyroid gland itself and malfunctions due to other causes, such as a tumor affecting the pituitary gland. (See **THYROID FUNCTION TESTS**.)

57 URIC ACID

Measures the amount of uric acid, a waste product, that, for the most part, is excreted by the kidneys. High blood levels are associated with *gout*, a painful but not dangerous inflammatory type of arthritis that usually affects the first joint in the big toe. High uric acid can also be a factor in *kidney stones*. A screening test for gout and kidney function often included in a multiple test panel.

58 VITAMIN B12 AND FOLIC ACID

Measures the blood level of these two vitamins essential for healthy red blood cells. Low levels can lead to *anemia* and can be caused by a *dietary deficiency, intestinal malabsorption* or *pernicious anemia*. Pernicious anemia is a condition in which vitamin B12 is present but can't be used by the body, because the stomach lacks a factor to absorb it. A screening test for *anemia*.

59 BONE MARROW ASPIRATION

The major components of your blood, red cells, white cells, and platelets all originate in your bone marrow. An analysis of bone marrow can provide important information concerning the health of the blood manufacturing process. It is particularly useful in cases of *anemia, leukemia,* other *cancers* that may have spread to the bone, and when tracking the effects of some toxic anti-cancer drugs. The sample is first suctioned and the cells are then examined under a microscope and analyzed by a pathologist and/or a hematologist. (The sample may also be cultured for bacteria.) It is much more revealing than a blood cell differential or **Complete Blood Count (CBC)**. However, because it can be a painful procedure, it is seldom ordered without strong cause.

The test is always performed by a doctor and is usually done in your hospital room a day after more simple blood tests have been performed. The sample is taken from the spongy marrow-filled bone of either the illiac crest (the back of the hip bone) or from the breast bone. (It is not unusual to receive a sedative a short time before the procedure.) After the area is cleaned and draped with sterile cloth, the skin and outer layer of bone are injected with a local anesthetic. You will feel the needle prick in the skin and a sharper pain and pressure as the bone is penetrated.

After the area is numb, the physician inserts a special needle (with a stylet for added strength) into the skin. You will feel pressure, pain and perhaps a twisting motion as the needle enters the marrow cavity. The stylet is quickly removed and replaced with a syringe. A little less than a teaspoon of marrow is drawn through the syringe. A technician in the room immediately prepares the sample on slides while the physician withdraws the needle and puts direct pressure on the puncture site for several minutes to prevent bleeding. He may push quite hard. You will be asked to lie still for a half hour, and the area will be checked for bleeding. The sample may be examined by a hematologist, specialist in the blood, and by an oncologist, a specialist in cancer. A full report takes at least a day.

Despite the sedative and local anesthetic, this test can make you howl, particularly while the marrow is being drawn up into the syringe. Patients have described feeling as if the bone had momentarily cracked. Fortunately the pain, like the whole procedure, is mercifully brief. Afterwards you may be tender for several days. A bruise at the puncture site may last as long as a week. A consent form is required.

60 BONE SCAN

A bone scan uses the techniques of nuclear medicine to create a picture of the bones, often revealing abnormalities much earlier than is

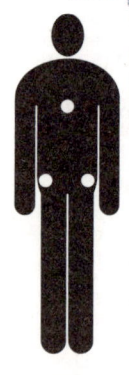

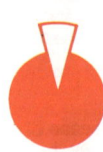

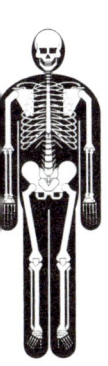

possible with conventional x-rays. In a nuclear scan, radionuclides (chemicals treated with minute amounts of radiation) are injected into the body. The particular chemical is chosen for its affinity to the specific organ under investigation. Once it is injected, it travels to and is absorbed by that organ. You are then scanned by a *gamma ray camera* which, like a geiger counter, measures the radiation emanating from you. This information is translated into a photo or diagram that can be read like an x-ray. By looking for spots of increased or decreased radiation absorption, defects can be identified.

No special preparation is needed for a bone scan. You go to the department of radiology or the nuclear medicine department, where the radionuclide is injected into a vein in your arm. This is no more painful than any other injection. Potassium is the chemical most often used. (It is essential for healthy bones and is typically absorbed by bone at a steady, predictable rate.) After the injection you will have to wait for up to 3 hours while the chemical is absorbed. During this time you may move around as you please. You will, however, be requested to drink lots of water, and right before the scan itself, you'll be asked to urinate. This rids the body of any extraneous radionuclide that hasn't been absorbed by the bone.

During the actual scanning you must lie still on an examining table for 30 to 60 minutes while the scanner moves over you. You may hear a clicking or buzzing sound. This is no cause for alarm. The scanner isn't exposing you to any more radiation. It is reading the minute amount of radiation that you are emitting.

Ideally, the scan reveals an even distribution of the radionuclide. Areas with heavy absorption (hot spots) may indicate *fractures, bone infection, arthritis* or *bone tumors*. Though the test is very sensitive—often revealing tumors 6 months earlier than is possible by x-ray—it is not very specific. A precise diagnosis of the bone abnormality cannot be made with a scan alone.

The test may be prescribed when diagnosing unexplained *bone pain,* when searching for *cancer* that may have spread to the bone, and when monitoring the effectiveness of cancer treatment. It is also used to locate the best site for biopsy and sometimes as a screening test for patients with *breast* or *prostate cancer*, both of which often spread to the bones.

The amount of radiation used in a bone scan is minute and is eliminated from the body within days. Total exposure is roughly equivalent to that received from a chest x-ray. However, the test is not recommended for pregnant or nursing mothers.

61 BRONCHOSCOPY

A fiberoptic device called a Bronchoscope allows a doctor to look inside the bronchi, the main air passageways of the lungs. The test is

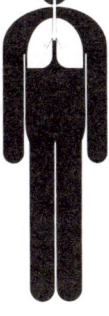

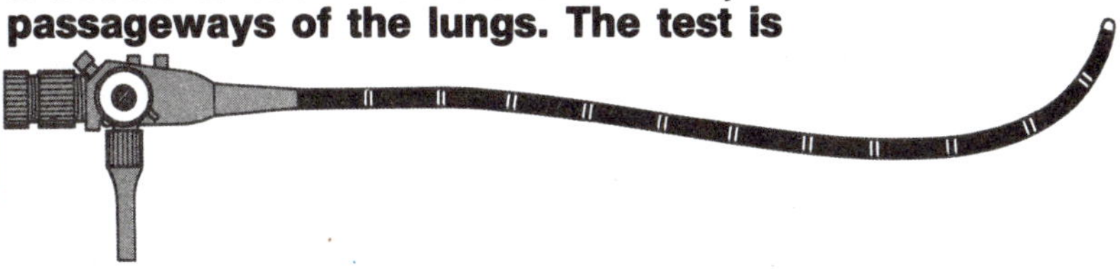

uncomfortable, and it can be a little scary, but it is not dangerous and can be important in diagnosing cancer and other diseases of the lung. While the doctor is looking at the lungs, he can use the bronchoscope to take samples of fluid and tissue for culture and biopsy.

It is typical for patients to receive several drugs before the procedure, including a sedative and something to reduce the urge to cough. The back of the throat is sprayed with a local anesthetic. The bronchoscope is then introduced, usually through the nose—this way the patient won't accidentally bite down on the delicate tube. Gradually the bronchoscope is threaded past the larynx (voice box) and down the trachea (wind pipe) into the bronchi. Each step of the way anesthetic is dripped through the tube of the bronchoscope numbing each area before the scope actually touches it. Usually the right bronchus is examined and then the left.

The bronchoscope has 2 bundles of fiberoptics—one to carry light, the other picture—and at least one hollow channel that runs the length of the scope. Fluids can be drawn up through the channel or drugs delivered through it. Areas obscured with blood or mucus can be washed with saline. A tiny cable operated whirring brush or forceps may be passed through to gather cell samples. A camera may be attached to the lense the doctor looks through and photos taken.

Before the test, a screening should be done for clotting and cardiovascular problems. You will be asked not to smoke for 24 hours before the test and not to eat or drink for 6 hours before the test. This is to avoid gagging and vomiting which could introduce foreign material into the lungs and lead to pneumonia.

With proper anesthesia you will probably experience discomfort but little pain. The biggest problem patients have is fear that air is being blocked and that they will suffocate. This is not true. Even with the bronchoscope in place, air flows easily in and out of the lungs. The best thing you can do is to relax as much as possible. This will also reduce the urge to cough.

You won't be allowed to eat or drink until the anesthesia wears off— usually in 2 hours. You may cough up a bit of blood-tinged sputum afterwards. A small amount is no cause for alarm.

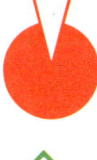

62 CARDIAC CATHETERIZATION CORONARY ANGIOGRAPHY, CORONARY ARTERIOGRAPHY, PULMONARY ANGIOGRAPHY

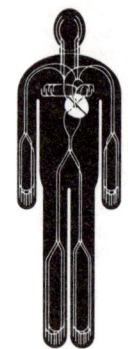

Cardiac Catheterization is probably the greatest technical advance in cardiology in the last 50 years. It's the celebrity of diagnostic tests, the most dramatic, the most expensive, and the final step in diagnosing a cardiac patient before the recommendation is made for or against heart surgery.

The procedure, which is done in a hospital, entails the insertion of one or more catheters (long, flexible, slender tubes) into an artery or vein and then guiding it until it enters the heart. Once in the heart the catheter can be used to take pressure readings, collect blood samples and inject dye that makes the chambers of the heart and the arteries that supply it with blood, visible on x-ray film. This detailed information, available no other way, can help diagnose narrowed or scarred heart valves, defects in the wall between heart chambers, the heart's overall ability to pump blood, and most commonly, *coronary artery disease*, which is a narrowing or blockage of the arteries that supply the heart itself with blood.

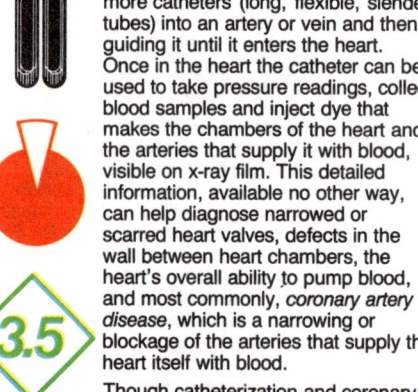

Though catheterization and coronary angiography have revolutionized the diagnosis of coronary artery disease, it is not a routine test but a test of the last resort to be performed after an **EKG, echocardiogram** and **exercise stress test**. It may reasonably be considered when a diagnosis of coronary artery disease is suspected but can't be proven, and a definite answer is important in planning a patient's therapy. Catheterization is also performed when heart failure or angina is uncontrollable medically and surgical treatment is seriously considered as an option. In this case it is essential because visualizing the coronary arteries tells the doctor which arteries if any have to be bypassed and whether the patient's heart is strong enough to survive surgery. Cardiac catheterization may also be justified for *cardiac neurotics*, people who have worked themselves up into a frenzy of fear about heart disease and who can only be calmed by x-rays that conclusively prove no disease is present. Catheterization should not be performed on patients who are known not to be good candidates for surgery.

Cardiac catheterization requires many of the precautions and preparations normally followed for surgery. Though it's becoming more and more common for patients to check into a hospital on the day of the procedure, many doctors prefer to check their patients in a day before when they go through a group of tests that may include a **complete blood count, electrolytes, SMA 6, prothrombin time, partial thromboplastin time**, and, perhaps as a precaution, **blood typing**.

You begin fasting after dinner on the night before the test. The following morning you are given a sedative, either orally or by injection. The attendant will make sure you've gone to the bathroom if you need to. Then you are wheeled into the cardiac catheterization lab.

This is a busy place. It contains an x-ray table, an overhead x-ray recorder, a television screen, several pieces of monitoring equipment and an emergency cart. Personnel include one or more doctors (cardiologists), one or more nurses, an x-ray technician and an electrical technician.

Because you will probably be awake during the entire procedure you are strapped to the table to prevent sudden movement. EKG leads will be attached to your wrists and ankles so your heart rate and rhythm can be monitored continuously, and an intravenous line may be started in your arm, in case any medication must be administered during the procedure. Peripheral room lights will probably be dimmed, both to help you relax and to help the doctors see the television screen which will show them the position of the catheter at all times.

The point of catheter insertion varies, but the most common point of entry is an artery or vein in the groin. The area is cleansed, draped and anesthetized with an injection. The injection stings but not terribly. Once the area is numb the blood vessel is either pierced directly or exposed with a very small incision. The catheter is then introduced and slowly moved towards your heart. Moving x-ray pictures shown on a television screen (flouroscopy) guide your doctor as the catheter is advanced. You may feel the catheter as it moves. It's a slightly uncomfortable, strange feeling, but not considered painful. Once the catheter reaches the heart, pressure readings from the various chambers are recorded and any blood samples needed are taken through the catheter. As the catheter moves through the heart it's not unusual to feel as though your heart skipped a beat or is beating abnormally fast. This is no cause for worry.

If you are undergoing the catheterization to assess *coronary artery disease* the doctor proceeds with coronary angiography. The catheter is maneuvered into the opening of a coronary artery and dye is released. You may feel an urge to cough and you will almost certainly feel a strong all-over flush and burning sensation. This can be quite strong and unpleasant, but it shouldn't last longer than 30 seconds. You may also have a metallic taste in your mouth and an urge to vomit. The moment the dye is released *cineangiograms* or x-ray movies are recorded on high speed film. The table you are on may be moved or tilted to allow several views and the catheter will probably be repositioned so that another coronary artery can be examined.

After the x-rays are taken the catheter is removed and direct pressure is put on the insertion site for 15-30 minutes. If an incision was made to expose the vein, it is closed with a few stitches. Typically you remain in the hospital for another day and will be kept in bed for the next 6 hours. You will want your rest. Most people find the test, which can take from 1 to 3 hours,

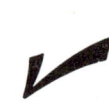

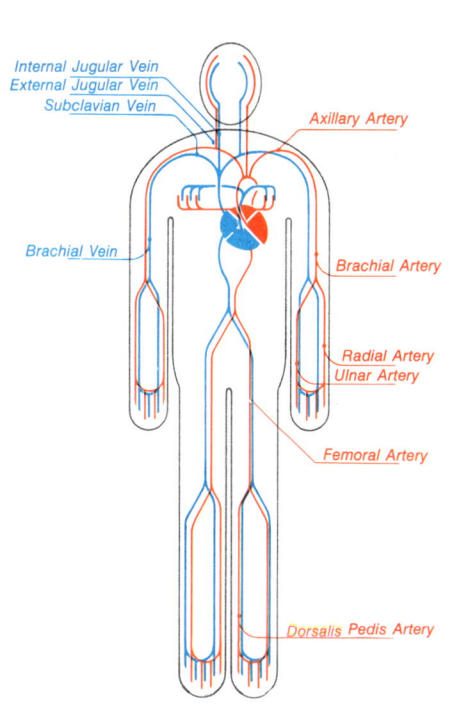

[Figure: diagram of human body showing vascular anatomy with labels: Internal Jugular Vein, External Jugular Vein, Subclavian Vein, Axillary Artery, Brachial Vein, Brachial Artery, Radial Artery, Ulnar Artery, Femoral Artery, Dorsalis Pedis Artery]

exhausting. During the first few hours your vital signs (pulse, respiration, temperature, and blood pressure) are checked frequently and the insertion site is checked for bleeding or swelling. You will be encouraged to drink plenty of fluids to help the kidneys excrete the dye, and you may be given fluids intravenously.

While it's clear that cardiac catheterization saves lives, it is not without risks. Approximately 1 in a thousand patients suffers a fatal heart attack during the procedure or within a day afterwards. There are also the risks of kidney damage from the dye, allergic reaction to the dye, and circulation problems arising at the puncture site.

Recent studies suggest that the procedure is over prescribed, and that some people are exposing themselves to risk unneccessarily. If your doctor suggests the procedure, make sure you get a full explanation of his or her reasons. Make sure that all other less invasive tests have been performed first. Since cardiac catheterization suggests the possibility of bypass surgery, bring this up in the discussion as well. Make sure that you really are a candidate for bypass surgery and that no other medical means exist to treat your symptoms. Lastly, don't be embarrassed about seeking a second opinion.

If you go ahead with the procedure, shop around for a good hospital. Though complications are really very infrequent you want to find a hospital with a well trained cardiac catheterization team that is prepared to deal with any emergency. Look for a hospital that performs at least 200 catheterizations a year.

CARDIAC CATHETERIZATION STUDIES

Pressure Readings. Pressure readings from the various chambers of the heart are transmitted from the tip of the catheter to a monitor in the catheterization lab. Differences in pressure from one side of a heart valve to the other can help diagnose a scarred or narrowed valve. Pressure readings also help assess the heart's overall ability to pump blood.

Blood Samples. The catheter is also used to take blood samples from the various chambers of the heart which are then analyzed for oxygen content. This can help detect leaks or defects in the wall that separates the heart chambers. For instance, if the blood that fills the right atrium has an oxygen content of 70 percent but the blood in the right ventricle has an oxygen content of 90 percent, it means that oxygen high blood must have leaked into the right ventricle from the left ventricle. These measurements can identify defects, and to some extent the percentages can be used to calculate the size of the defect and whether it needs surgical repair.

Coronary Angiography. Probably the most common reason cardiac catheterization is ordered. The catheter is inserted into an artery and guided up to the aorta, the huge blood vessel that receives all the heart's freshly oxygenated blood before it goes to the body. From the aorta the catheter is guided to the openings of the coronary arteries and dye is injected. The coronary arteries are the arteries that supply the heart muscle itself with the blood it needs to live. Any blockage or narrowing should show up very clearly on the x-rays taken right after the dye injection. If there is severe blockage of these arteries surgery may be considered.

Left Heart Angiography. The catheter may be withdrawn from the coronary arteries and threaded through the left atrium into the left ventricle where a large amount of dye is injected and more x-ray movies taken. These x-rays or *ventriculograms* help the cardiologist detect abnormal motion characteristic of weakened or scarred muscle wall. By carefully examining how much dye is pumped out of the ventricle during successive heart beats the *ejection fraction* can be calculated. This is the percentage of the blood that is pumped out of the left ventricle with each beat. In a normal heart about 60 percent of the ventricular blood is pumped out. In a diseased failing heart 30 percent or less may be pumped. The ejection fraction is a critically important determination of which patients will be able to survive surgery.

Pulmonary Angiography. A catheter is inserted in a vein and guided through the right side of the heart until it reaches the pulmonary arteries, the blood vessels that carry blood to the lungs. Dye is injected and x-rays taken that reveal the structure of and any abnormalities in the arteries that supply the lungs. Most often used to detect a pulmonary embolism (blood clot) a potentially very dangerous condition where part of a lung is deprived of blood and oxygen. This in turn puts a great strain on the left side of the heart. Diagnosis of pulmonary embolism is one of the few instances in which cardiac catheterization may be done on an emergency basis.

63 CARDIAC ENZYMES — HEART ENZYMES

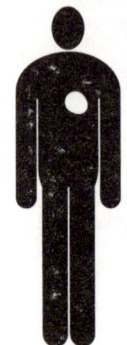

If your heart has been damaged (as in a heart attack), several enzymes found inside the cells of the heart will leak into the bloodstream. An analysis of the blood level of these enzymes can be very useful—along with a careful physical exam and an **EKG**—in determining if someone admitted to the hospital with chest pain and other symptoms of heart attack, has actually had one. If there has been a heart attack, cardiac enzyme studies can help determine when it took place and how much of the heart muscle has been damaged. It is probably the most common test after EKG for diagnosing heart attack.

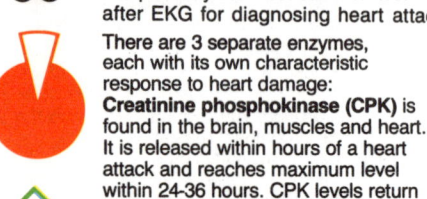

There are 3 separate enzymes, each with its own characteristic response to heart damage:
Creatinine phosphokinase (CPK) is found in the brain, muscles and heart. It is released within hours of a heart attack and reaches maximum level within 24-36 hours. CPK levels return to normal within 2-3 days. **Serum glutamic-oxaloacetic transaminase (SGOT)** is found primarily in the heart and liver. It is released within 6-10 hours after a heart attack and reaches maximum level 1-2 days later. SGOT returns to near normal within 5 days.
Lactic dehydrogenase (LDH) is found in red blood cells, muscle, liver and heart. Released within 24-72 hours after a heart attack, LDH reaches maximum level within 2-4 days and returns to normal in 10-14 days. It is particularly useful in late diagnosis of heart attack.

Damage to other organs, such as the liver or brain, will also result in elevated levels of 1 or 2 of these enzymes. In a heart attack, however, levels of all 3 enzymes will rise and fall in a predictable pattern. Thus, heart attack diagnosis is based on the comparative analysis of all 3 enzymes over time. Someone in the hospital for observation after a known or suspected heart attack, may have blood taken several times a day over the course of several days. All 3 enzymes can be analyzed from a single blood sample.

If the results of cardiac enzyme study are not conclusive because of possible damage elsewhere in the body, more complex blood tests called *isoenzyme studies* can be done to isolate and measure the enzyme released by the heart.

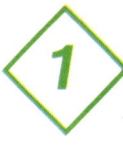

64 CARDIAC SCAN

Cardiac scanning is a low risk, highly accurate technique used to determine whether or not a heart attack has occurred, and if so, its location and severity.

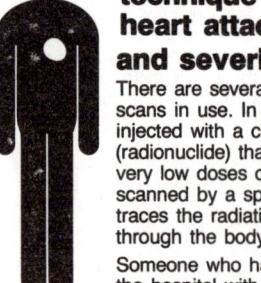

There are several types of cardiac scans in use. In every case you're injected with a chemical (radionuclide) that's been exposed to very low doses of radiation, and then scanned by a special camera that traces the radiation as it passes through the body.

Someone who has been rushed to the hospital with chest pain and other heart attack symptoms will probably be given an **Electrocardiogram** and have blood drawn for **Cardiac Enzymes** studies, but these more common tests may not always be enough to determine whether the patient has actually had a heart attack. In such a case, a cardiac scan may yield a definitive answer and help locate the precise area and size of the heart attack. Though the equipment is usually located at a hospital, you needn't check in to be tested. There are 3 major types of heart scan:

Hot spot imaging. You receive an injection of radioactive pyrophosphate. Thirty to 60 minutes later, when the chemical has been absorbed into the heart muscle, you will be asked to lie still on the examining table while a scanning camera moves over you. The camera registers the radionuclide distribution pattern and translates the information into a picture. Areas with increased radionuclide activity indicate heart attack. This type of scan can make a definitive diagnosis within 24-48 hours after a heart attack, sometimes even sooner. The actual scanning takes about 15 minutes. It is painless and there are no aftereffects.
Thallium Scan. (cold spot imaging). This scan shows which areas of heart muscle are not receiving enough oxygen. In most cases it is done in conjunction with an **Exercise Stress Test**. You may be asked to fast for several hours before going to the nuclear medicine lab, where electrocardiogram leads will be attached to your chest and a blood pressure cuff put on your arm. In some cases an intravenous lead will be started in your arm. Once the preparation is complete, you exercise, under supervision, on a stationary bicycle or a treadmill. You do this for 10 to 30 minutes, until it is determined that maximum exertion has been reached. At this point thallium (a radioactive chemical) is injected or infused through the intravenous lead, and you are led to an examining table where you must remain still while the scanning is done. Areas of the heart receiving insufficient blood and oxygen will show decreased thallium absorption. The test is useful in detecting deprived areas of heart muscle that are at risk for heart attack as well as areas that have already suffered an attack in the past. It is also useful in evaluating the heart's pumping ability. There are no aftereffects associated with the test other than tiredness. It should not, however, be performed on any patient who wouldn't be considered for a stress electrocardiogram.

Blood Pool Scan. Red blood cells are labeled with a radioactive compound and injected into a vein in the arm. Scanning of the blood as it moves through the heart is done in synchronization with an **Electrocardiogram**. This gives the physician precise information on how effectively the heart is moving blood. Some of the radioactive material also penetrates heart muscle which may allow the physician to observe the heart wall in motion, information that otherwise is only available through **Cardiac Catheterization**, a more expensive, painful and risky procedure.

Heart scans are probably used to rule out a diagnosis as often as to confirm one. If, for instance, a patient has chest pain and a questionable EKG but a negative heart scan, the physician can rule out heart attack as the source of pain and thus avoid more invasive testing. Heart scans are also used to evaluate patients before and after bypass surgery.

65 COMPUTERIZED AXIAL TOMOGRAPHY CAT/CT SCAN

Computerized axial tomography or CAT scan, is a highly sophisticated form of x-ray, 100 times as sensitive as an ordinary x-ray, which

takes a cross-sectional view of the head or body.

The CAT scanner which looks something like a giant doughnut in a box, is usually located in a special radiology room in a hospital. During an exam, you lie on a flat movable table inside the hole of the scanner. Inside and to one side of the scanner ring is an x-ray tube, and opposite that, receptors which detect radiation. These rotate around your head or body in a 360-degree arc, taking thousands of variable depth x-ray readings which are then interpreted by a computer in an adjacent room and converted into video or Polaroid images.

A CAT scan image shows the size and shape of body organs, layer by layer, in a kind of horizontal slicing. It's much like looking at the rings in the trunk of a tree. Because the CAT scanner can distinguish between even slight variations in tissue density, it's extremely useful in diagnosing diseases and injuries of the head; in fact, the first CAT scanners developed in the early 1970s were used only for cranial studies. Since 1976, however, the development of large scanners has allowed for examinations of various parts of the body. These images are particularly accurate in identifying *tumors, blood clots, cysts, hemorrhage, liver* and *kidney disease* and certain *diseases of the spine and large blood vessels.*

There are 2 types of CAT scanners: one allows the entire body to be moved inside the cylinder. The other, smaller model is only used to examine the head.

Body Scan. Preparation for a CAT scan is minimal. No hospitalization is required. Certain abdominal scans require a short fast and/or an enema to clear the bowel of feces and gas. Occasionally a sedative is administered before the procedure to help you relax and stay still during the study.

Before the test begins, you remove part or all of your clothing and put on a hospital gown. Certain body scans, particularly those that focus on the liver or kidneys, may require the use of a contrast dye to make the soft tissue more visible on the x-ray film. The dye may be administered orally or rectally before scanning, or by injection during the scan. If you receive the dye by injection you may feel a brief all-over flush and burning sensation accompanied by nausea and a metallic taste in the mouth.

You are positioned comfortably on the table with a strap holding you in place. While the pictures are being taken, you will hear the clicking sounds of gears and motors inside the ring as the x-ray equipment rotates around you. You may be asked to hold your breath from time to time. Though it's difficult, it's important to remain still; any movement will blur the image.

The table moves you forward until you are surrounded by the huge machine, but not shut off completely—there is light inside. You'll also be able to talk to the examiner if you wish, through a 2-way intercom. The CAT scan equipment is kept cool, about the temperature of a normally air-conditioned room, so you may want to request a blanket.

Head Scan. The procedure for a head scan is identical to a body scan, except that only the head is placed inside the hole of the scanner, which has a cradle-like depression that fits you like a rubber helmet. Your head is held in place gently but securely by a strap. All objects are removed from your hair, and it is combed to lie smoothly around your head. Your face is not covered or blocked. You must remain stationary during the scanning. Even talking or sighing may distort the image.

A CAT scan, head or body, takes less than an hour. Afterwards, you can resume your normal activities and diet.

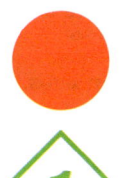

Except for having to keep your body or head absolutely still—*a real pain in the neck,* as some have described it—undergoing a CAT scan is generally quite painless. Since an extremely narrow x-ray beam is focused on the body, the total amount of x-ray exposure is less than standard x-rays. If dye will be used inform your doctor of any allergies, particularly to iodine or seafood which is high in iodine. An allergic reaction to the contrast dye is the only possible side effect and this can be avoided if you inform your physician about all allergies.

66 CHEST X-RAY

A chest x-ray, also called a plain film or a flat plate, is the most frequently performed x-ray, accounting for 50 percent of all x-ray studies

performed. It is probably a bit overused but it is extraordinarily useful, providing a look at the ribs, lungs and heart.

No special preparation is needed for the study, which takes place in the radiology department of a hospital or in your doctor's office. You are asked to undress from the waist up and remove any jewelry. Women may be given a gown to wear. You stand with your chest next to a photographic plate while the technician positions you and explains that you must stay still and briefly hold your breath while the x-ray is being taken. Before the x-ray is taken you should be given a lead apron which protects your reproductive organs from stray radiation. If one isn't offered, ask for it. The technician will briefly retreat to another room or behind a partition while the x-ray is taken. You are then repositioned and a side view taken. The film should be available the same day. Usually a radiologist looks at the picture and prepares a report which is forwarded to your own doctor along with the film.

A chest x-ray may be ordered for any patient with *shortness of breath, chest pain, wheezing* or a particularly *bad cough* that brings up phlegm. Though the study can yield important information on a variety of diseases, the most common reason for an x-ray is to rule out or confirm *pneumonia*. X-rays pass through normal air-filled lung tissue which shows up black on x-rays. In pneumonia the inflamed tissue shows up white. After treatment, another chest x-ray is frequently taken to see if the area has shrunk or vanished. Other conditions which may be investigated by a chest x-ray include:

Pulmonary embolism (blood clot in the lung). Helps identify size, location and amount of tissue damaged by the clot.

Congestive heart failure. Helps determine if the heart is unhealthily enlarged and whether there is fluid in the lungs.

Bronchitis and **Emphysema.** Used to determine the severity of these diseases. Usually by the time either is visible on an x-ray, some irreversible damage has been done.

Asthma. Primarily done to see if pneumonia, a possible complication of asthma, is present.

Cancer. Used in locating a mass in the lungs or one pressing on them from the outside. Not particularly useful as a screening test since lung cancer is usually well established by the time it shows up on an x-ray.

When tuberculosis was more of a problem than it is today, chest x-rays were common screening tests performed on every patient entering the hospital. While they are no longer recommended as screening tests, because of the dangers of radiation, these statistics may help put the minimal risk in perspective. Radiation dosage is measured in milliroentgens or mr's. The average radiation exposure you get just from living in the world, that is underneath the ultraviolet rays of the sun and above the uranium 238 in the soil, comes to 100mr a year. A chest x-ray exposes you to 20mrs. The exposure from scattered radiation to your reproductive organs from an x-ray is 0.04mr in men and 0.2mr in women. In other words, it would take 2500 x-rays for a man or 500 for a woman to equal the radiation exposure your reproductive organs receive in a year of living.

67 CHLAMYDIA

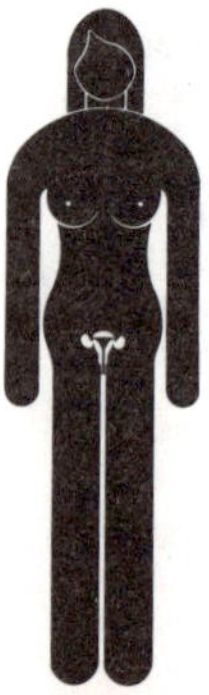

Topping the charts with 3 to 10 million cases a year, chlamydia is clearly the most common sexually transmitted disease of the decade.

Ironically, few people have ever heard of it. Until recently chlamydia was difficult to identify in a lab; it is likely that more than half of what used to be diagnosed as *non-specific urethritis* or *non-gonoccocal urethritis* were actually cases of chlamydia. Furthermore, a large number of difficult to diagnose cases of *vaginitis* and *pelvic inflammatory disease (PID)* are probably caused by chlamydia as well.

Though easily treatable, the disease is insidious because symptoms are slow to appear, often mild and in some cases fail to appear at all. Many cases go undiagnosed or may be diagnosed as gonorrhea, which is a simple mistake to make, since 30-40 percent of those with gonorrhea also have chlamydia. Untreated chlamydia can have very unpleasant consequences. In men, the disease begins as an infection of the urethra, but it can spread to the testicles and cause *sterility*. In women, the infection can spread from the vagina or cervix to the fallopian tubes, eventually causing *scarring*. Scarred fallopian tubes may make it impossible to conceive or increase the possibility of *tubal pregnancy*. Chlamydia is now implicated as the initial cause in 50-90 percent of all cases of *pelvic inflammatory disease (PID)*, a dangerous and painful condition that may result in female sterility. A baby born to a woman with chlamydia is at high risk for developing *conjunctivitis*,

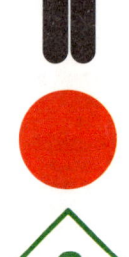

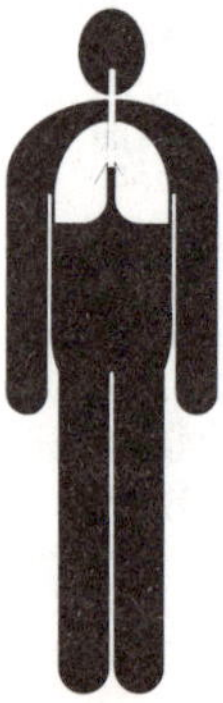

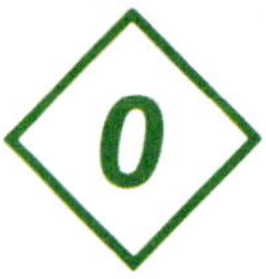

1

an eye infection that may lead to blindness.

On the plus side, once it has been diagnosed, chlamydia is easy to cure. Treatment consists of a long course, 7 to 21 days, of antibiotics, tetracyclines or sulfonamides taken orally. Penicillin, commonly given to treat gonorrhea, is not adequate. However, because of the rise of chlamydia, more and more cases of gonorrhea are being treated initially with tetracyclines in hope of knocking out any chlamydia infection as well. If you are being treated for chlamydia, it is essential that your partner(s) be treated as well. Even if they show no symptoms of infection, chances are they have it and will only end up reinfecting you. (Some doctors refer to this as the *ping pong* effect.)

There are 2 testing methods used to diagnose chlamydia. A culture is the older, better known method, but even so, it is a difficult test to perform correctly and may only be available at hospitals, the larger labs and VD clinics. The sample is taken the same way as the sample for gonorrhea. A cotton tipped applicator is inserted in the vagina or tip of the penis. A sample of bacteria-filled discharge is obtained, cultured and examined for bacterial growth. The results take from 3-5 days and the test is expensive. A lab will probably charge twice the price of a standard vaginal culture and a hospital may charge 4 times as much. A newer method is MicroTrak. Although not widely available at present, it is likely to become more common because it is very inexpensive and results are available within a day. Sampling technique is basically the same as above. However, because the test requires infected cells rather than just discharge, the sample taking is a bit rougher and stings a bit more than usual.

Symptoms in both men and women are similar to those for gonorrhea. There may be a slight cloudy discharge and pain on urination, as well as an urge to urinate often. Women may experience pain during intercourse, fever and lower abdominal pain.

Up to 10 percent of all college students have chlamydia.

Chlamydia
Number of cases in US, 1984

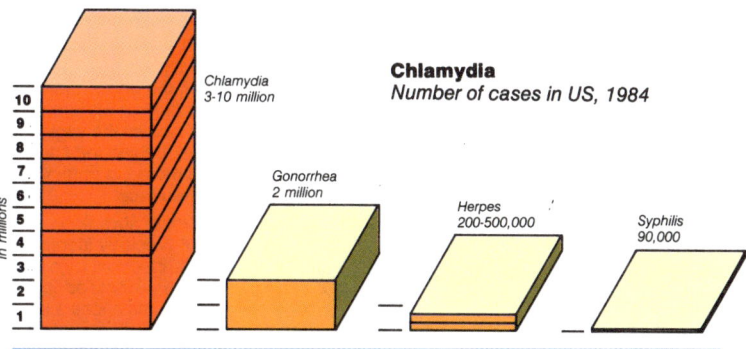

- Chlamydia 3-10 million
- Gonorrhea 2 million
- Herpes 200-500,000
- Syphilis 90,000

68 COLONOSCOPY ENDOSCOPY

Tremendous technical progress during the last 20 years in the field of fiberoptics has now made it relatively simple for your physician to view the entire large intestine (about 58 inches from rectum to cecum) without surgery.

The tool that makes this possible is the colonoscope, essentially a long flexible telescope about as thick as your index finger. Inside it, thousands of fine glass threads are grouped into 2 sets of fiberoptic bundles. One set carries light down the length of the tube to deep in the bowel, while the other set carries an image from the bowel to the eyepiece your physician looks through. Typically, a colonoscope has 2 other small channels. One is used to inflate the bowel with air or suction off secretions. Tiny cable-operated instruments can be passed through the other channel to retrieve tissue for analysis (**Biopsy**) or to remove polyps.

Colonoscopy is performed when *severe pain, diarrhea* or *gastrointestinal bleeding* persists and cannot be investigated by any less invasive procedure. It may also be ordered to more closely examine or remove irregularities that have shown up in a **Barium enema** study. The information gathered from the exam is used in diagnosing *ulcerative colitis, inflammatory bowel disease, cancer* and other conditions.

Because the bowel must be clear of fecal matter for the doctor to see the intestinal lining, you will be restricted to a clear liquid diet (which includes broth, jello, coffee, tea and juices, but no solid food and no milk products) for 48 hours before the test. The night before the test, you will be given laxatives and then prohibited from eating after midnight. Some doctors order an enema early the next morning.

The decision about sedation is made by you and your physician. Though it is not absolutely necessary, it is common to receive valium or demerol through an intravenous line. The object of sedation is to relax you, not to put you under, for often your cooperation is needed.

Once sedation is complete, you lie on your left side with your knees drawn up and the sterile gown or drapes slightly parted. The doctor lubricates your anus and the scope and gently begins insertion. Although the position may be embarrassing and the feeling unusual and uncomfortable, it is not particularly painful. Deep slow breathing through the mouth helps you relax and reduces the urge to go to the bathroom.

After the first several inches, insertion is completed under direct observation.

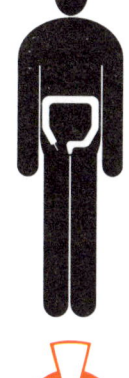

Because the colon bends and folds, the physician may ask you to shift position to allow further penetration of the scope. Air is often forced through the colonoscope to inflate the bowel, making insertion and viewing easier. It may cause a cramping feeling, not unlike gas pains.

Once the scope is entirely inserted, it is very slowly withdrawn while the doctor looks at the lining of the bowel for any abnormalities. Frequently colonoscopes have a spare viewing line for students. Many physicians are willing to hook it up so you can get a look too. At this time a cable-controlled brush or forceps may be inserted in the scope and a tissue sample taken.

You may feel a slight tugging, but chances are you won't feel anything at all. Within an hour the scope is withdrawn and the exam completed. The combination of the exam, the fasting and the cleansing procedure can be exhausting. You'll probably want to rest for a moment on the table before returning home or to your room. If the test is done on an outpatient basis, you should have someone drive you home. Unless the doctor specifies otherwise, you can resume a normal diet immediately, though you will be encouraged to drink extra fluids to make up for dehydration caused by laxatives. Many people find a warm bath very soothing after colonoscopy.

69 COLPOSCOPY

Colposcopy may be the first test ordered after abnormal findings in a Pap smear. It allows the physician to get an extremely detailed look inside the vagina and the cervix. The goal is to identify exactly where the abnormal cells are located so they can be more directly sampled. In some cases colposcopy may reduce the need for **biopsy**, a procedure that could require hospitalization.

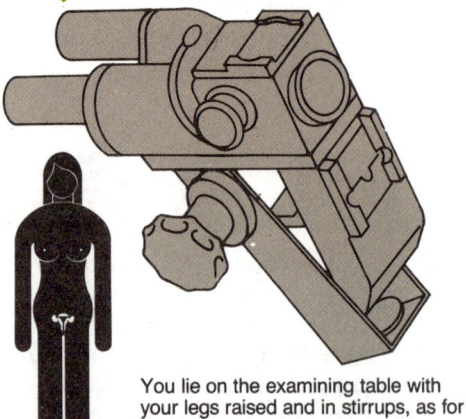

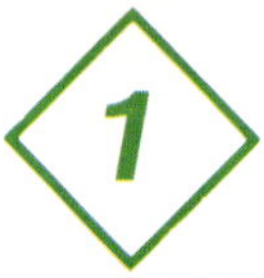

You lie on the examining table with your legs raised and in stirrups, as for a regular pelvic examination. The physician inserts a speculum into the vagina which spreads the vaginal walls and provides a clear field of vision. The vagina and cervix are cleaned with cotton balls or a sterile solution, which removes the normal mucus secretions. A cell sampling, like a **Pap smear**, may be taken at this time as well. Then the colposcope is placed at the vaginal opening and focused on the back of the vaginal wall. The colposcope, essentially a microscope with its own light source and extra lenses that allow it to focus closely on distant objects, never actually enters the vagina. During the exam the doctor may rotate the speculum or withdraw it very slowly. This causes the vaginal walls to close slowly behind the speculum and allows for a more thorough viewing of their surface.

The main advantage of colposcopy is that it precisely identifies the location of the abnormal area that was only indirectly identified in the Pap smear. In some instances a tissue sample will be taken with small tweezers or a curette during the procedure. Some discomfort is associated with the sampling, but nothing requiring even local anesthesia. There are no aftereffects unless a sample was taken, in which case there may be light bleeding. If bleeding is heavy, report to your doctor. Colposcopy, which can be performed in the hospital or in your gynecologist's office takes about 15 minutes. The doctor may be able to discuss his findings with you immediately but lab results from tissue samples usually take about 3 days.

70 CREATININE CLEARANCE TEST

Creatinine Clearance is one of the most accurate gauges of kidney function. It is a combination test performed on urine samples collected over a 24-hour period and 1 blood sample. Both are measured for creatinine, a metabolic waste product that is filtered from the blood by the kidneys.

Kidneys function as strainers, cleansing the bloodstream of wastes such as creatinine while preserving those chemicals that the body needs. However, a waste product is never completely removed from the blood in 1 pass through the kidneys. About 5 pints of blood pass through the kidneys every minute, but only a fraction of that can be filtered at a time. By comparing the amount of creatinine in the blood with the amount excreted in urine over 24 hours, your doctor figures out the kidneys' *clearance rate* which means the amount of blood that is cleaned over a set period of time. The clearance rate shows how well the kidney is doing its job.

To begin the test, you empty your bladder and note the time. All urine passed over the next 24 hours will be saved and analyzed. At some point during those 24 hours, a standard blood sample is drawn. This test is almost always ordered in conjunction with a **Blood Urea Nitrogen** test. It is commonly recommended for people with known or suspected kidney disease, or to measure the extent of dehydration when there has been severe vomiting or diarrhea.

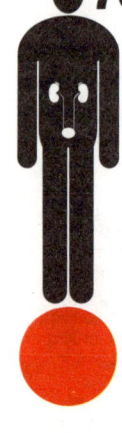

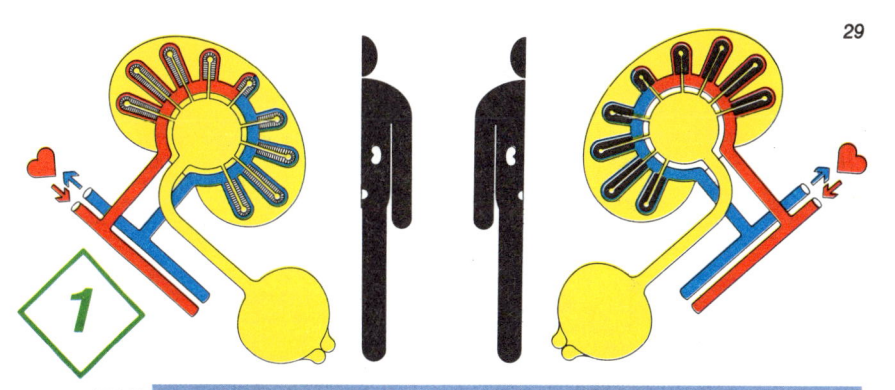

71 CYSTOSCOPY

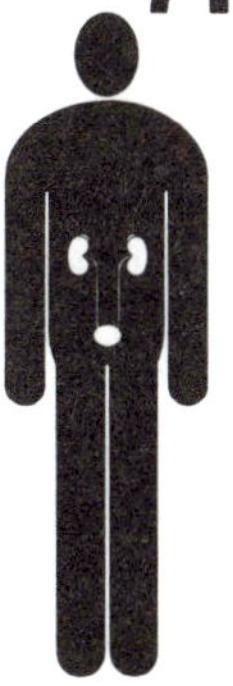

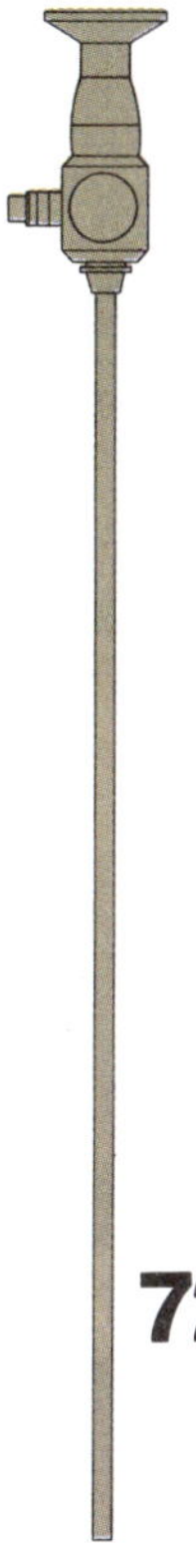

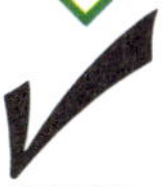

This procedure used to be painful and frightening, but modern techniques, including smaller scopes, local numbing agents and good sedation, have considerably reduced discomfort and anxiety. In many cases cystoscopy can be done on an outpatient basis in either a hospital cystoscopy suite or a urologist's office.

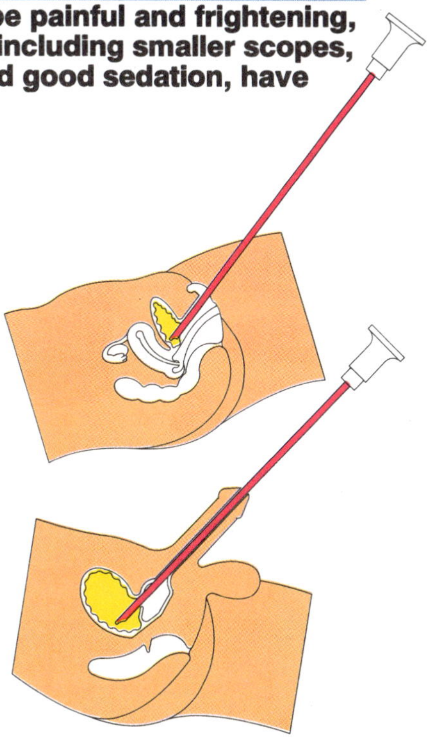

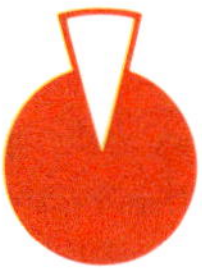

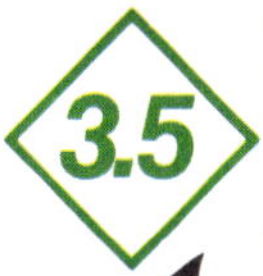

The physician uses a cystoscope, a rigid metal tube with lenses and a fiberoptic light source to look inside the urethra and bladder and examine the ureters. In males, cystoscopy may also be used to examine the prostate gland. *Tumors* and *stones* may be detected, as well as the cause of *urinary pain, bleeding* and *chronic bladder infection*. In addition, catheters can be inserted through the cystoscope into the ureters. This allows for direct, sterile sampling of urine from one specific kidney or the other, a potentially important diagnostic aid where kidney disease is suspected. In some cases small instruments can be passed through the scope and used to remove stones and small bladder tumors.

You may be told to avoid solid foods the morning of the test and will certainly be told to drink plenty of fluids. This increases urine flow which reduces the risk of infection and makes urine sampling easier. Sedation (valium or demerol) is started an hour before the examination. (Some patients need general anesthesia, in which case the test is done in a hospital, requires fasting after midnight and probably intravenous fluids.)

Once in the cystoscopy suite you lie on an examining table with your legs in stirrups. You're draped with sterile cloth and the penis or vagina is thoroughly cleansed. A local anesthetic is instilled in the urethra; this stings briefly. When the area is numb you will be asked to remain very still as the lubricated cystoscope is slowly inserted in the urethra and from there into the bladder. This can be quite uncomfortable and is accompanied by an urge to urinate.

The exam lasts about 20 minutes. When it is over, you will be asked to rest for a moment on the examining table before returning to your room. If the cystoscopy was conducted under local anesthesia, you will often be permitted to go home immediately but you should have someone else do the driving. Attention will be paid to your ability to urinate. It is usual for urination to be slightly painful at first and the urine tinted pink with blood. If blood is heavy or pain extreme, your doctor must be informed. If after several hours you are unable to urinate, a catheter may be inserted to assist you. Urine flow is critically important in avoiding infection. Other aftereffects may include back pain and bladder spasms. A warm bath and high fluid intake may be recommended to ease your discomfort.

Rarely, the urethra or bladder may be perforated during cystoscopy. A more common complication is infection. Antibiotics are often prescribed for several days after the exam as a protective measure.

72 DOPPLER ULTRASOUND

Doppler ultrasound is a noninvasive technique used to analyze moving structures within the body, in particular the movement of blood within

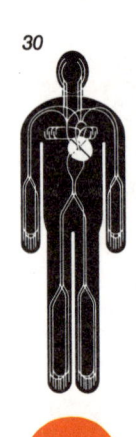

arteries and veins. A small handheld instrument called a transducer is placed against the skin, above the blood vessel in question. High frequency soundwaves are reflected back from the blood vessel to the transducer which amplifies them so they can be heard through earphones worn by the examiner. The *pitch* of the returning soundwaves is proportional to the velocity of the moving blood. This is called the Doppler effect. It is the same principle that makes the sound of a moving train whistle suddenly sound lower after the train passes you. The sound of blood moving through healthy arteries is a loud swish. In diseased or obstructed arteries the noise is low and muffled, in blocked arteries no sound is heard at all. Blood vessels in the arm, calf, thigh, ankle and neck are all commonly checked with Doppler ultrasound. There is no pain or discomfort associated with the study. The examiner dabs a bit of oil or jelly to help make good contact and then puts the transducer on the skin. In some cases, several blood vessels may be checked and the exact placement of the transducer may be marked on the skin with an indelible marker for later reference.

The test is particularly useful in assessing patients with swollen or sensitive limbs who may have a *blood clot* or who have *thrombophlebitis,* a disease where the deep veins of the leg become inflamed and narrowed. It may also be used on *stroke* patients to detect obstructions in the arteries that supply the brain. A handheld Doppler ultrasound device is also used to take blood pressure measurements in babies or people with extremely low blood pressure. The same type of equipment is also used to detect the motion of an unborn baby's beating heart. (See **Fetal Monitoring**.)

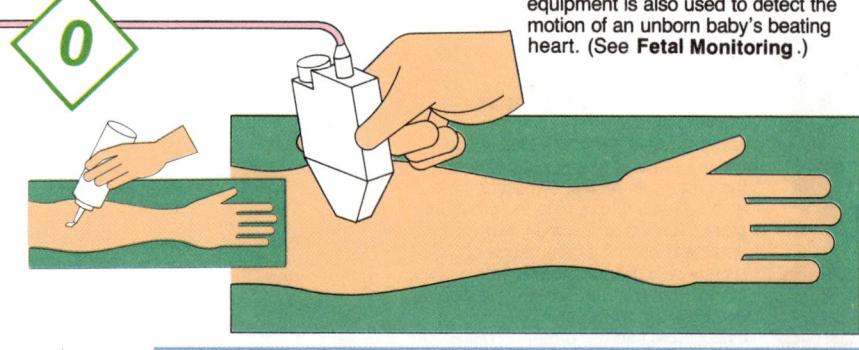

73 ECHOCARDIOGRAM CARDIAC ECHO, ECHOGRAM

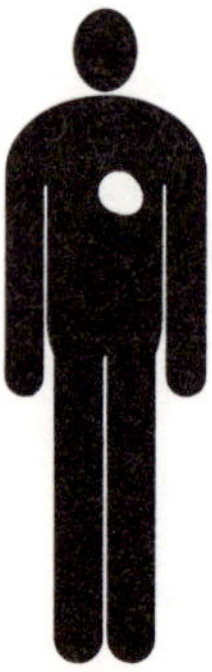

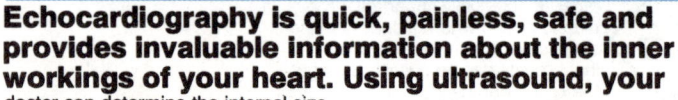

Echocardiography is quick, painless, safe and provides invaluable information about the inner workings of your heart. Using ultrasound, your doctor can determine the internal size of the heart chambers, the thickness of the chamber walls, whether there is excess fluid building up around the heart, contractibility of the heart muscle and whether the 4 valves of the heart are narrowed or leaking. High frequency soundwaves (much higher than can be heard by the human ear), are beamed at the heart from the tip of a *transducer,* a small handheld instrument that looks like a microphone. Some of the soundwaves are reflected back to the transducer which converts them to electrical signals and sends them to the echocardiograph machine. The machine translates the signals into visual information, either a graph or a picture, that can be shown on a monitor—much the same way underwater sonar or aerial radar is displayed.

There are 2 basic echocardiograph modes. Your doctor's machinery may do one or the other, or frequently both at the same time. In *M-Mode,* the information is presented in a graphic wave format that must be read almost like an **EKG** report. (See **74**.) A *real-time,* or *2D,* echocardiogram, turns the signal into pictorial information, a black and white slice or cross section of your heart, where all the internal contours are discernible. A series of these images is taken in rapid succession and recorded on videotape, making a movie of the inside of your heart.

Though the test may be performed in a hospital, an increasing number of internists and cardiologists have their own equipment and perform the test, with the aid of a technician, in their offices. No special preparation is required. You will undress from the waist up and lie down on an examining table. In most cases an Electrocardiogram is done at the same time, so several electrodes will be painlessly placed on your chest and/or your wrists and ankles. A small amount of gel or mineral oil will be spread on your chest to help conduct sound without interference from the air. The technician will then take the transducer and place it on your chest in a space between the ribs. The room lights are usually dimmed so the TV monitor can be seen more easily. While the technician looks for the best viewing points, you may be asked to turn and lie on your left side. When a good spot is found, you will be asked to remain still while the transducer is slowly tilted from side to side. The exam should be over in a half hour, perhaps a bit longer if visualization is difficult. (This can happen if the patient is obese or has a large barrel-shaped chest.) If a technician performs the test, a doctor may briefly review the tape to make sure the necessary information is there. You will then be allowed to leave.

In general, an echocardiogram is ordered after a less expensive EKG, but before a more expensive **Nuclear cardiac scan**.(see **64**), and the much more expensive and invasive **Cardiac catheterization** study (See **62**.) When it is available, an echocardiogram is

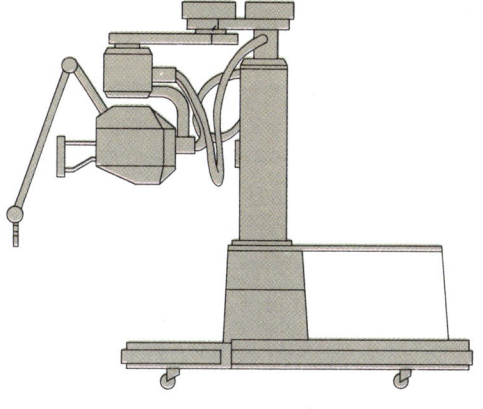

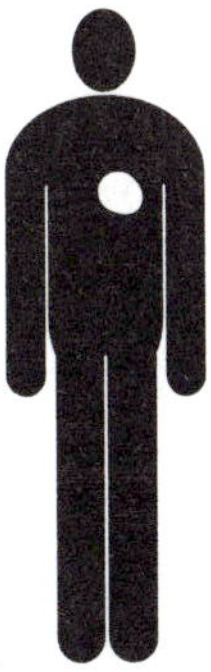

31

to show an enlarged heart. Not only is it more accurate than x-rays, it is also safer. There is absolutely no radiation exposure to patient or operator from ultrasound.

Echocardiography is particularly good at identifying malfunctioning heart valves and the abnormal enlargement of heart chambers that often result when the heart is forced to work harder to make up for the inefficient valve. Heart valve abnormalities often make very recognizable murmurs or clicks that can be heard through a stethoscope. If your personal physician has heard such a noise, he may order an echocardiogram before ordering the more common electrocardiogram.

also preferred over **Chest x-rays,** which have conventionally been used

74 ELECTROCARDIOGRAM ECG, CARDIOGRAM, EKG, 12-LEAD EKG, HOLTER MONITOR

Like a car engine, the heart depends on electrical energy to start it and keep it beating regularly. This energy is generated by the body's own

pacemaker, a tiny bundle of nerve fibers called the *sinoatrial (SA) node,* which is located in the upper right chamber or atrium of the heart. In a healthy heart, the impulse follows a strict rhythmic pattern. The impulse is fired and sends an electric wave to the 2 upper chambers, the atria. They contract and force the blood into the larger lower chambers, the ventricles.

The wave of electricity then moves to the *atrioventricular (AV) node,* the junction where the signal is split and conducted to the 2 ventricles; the ventricles contract and pump blood to the lungs and the body. There is a brief period of relaxation as the atria fill with returning blood and the SA node prepares to fire again. Then the whole process is repeated—usually about 2 times a second.

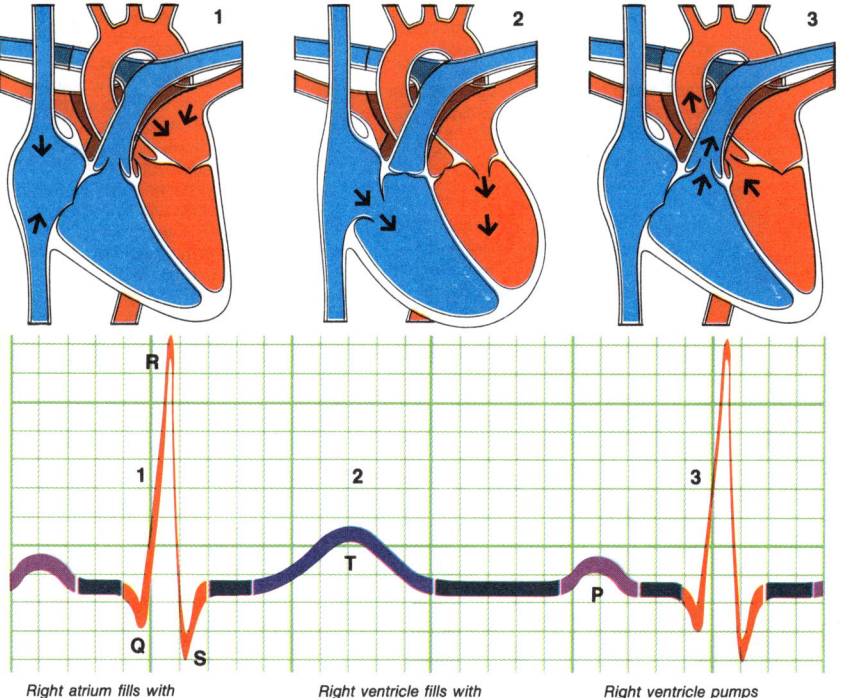

Right atrium fills with deoxygenated venous blood
Left atrium fills with oxygenated blood from the lungs

Right ventricle fills with deoxygenated blood
Left ventricle fills with oxygenated blood

Right ventricle pumps blood to lungs
Left ventricle pumps blood to body

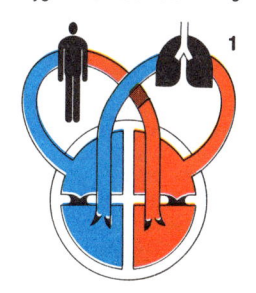

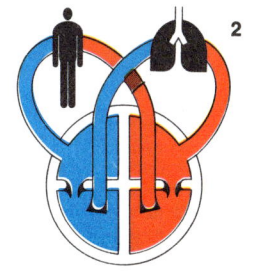

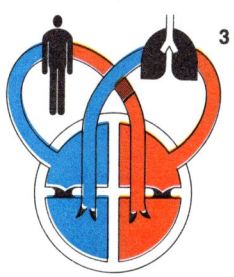

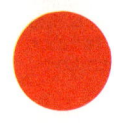

An electrocardiogram measures the pattern of this electric wave as it moves through the heart muscle.

The test, which is painless, non-invasive and over in about 15 minutes, has become a fundamental part of cardiac diagnosis. It is performed almost as a matter of course when someone presents any of the symptoms of *heart disease,* which might include *shortness of breath, chest pain, palpitations, dizziness* or *faintness.* For those over 40, it may be a routine part of a complete physical. In the hospital, an EKG is almost always performed as a screening test before surgery. While there seems to be no compelling need for regular EKGs if you are under 40, have no family history of heart disease and normal blood pressure, your doctor still may recommend at least 1 baseline EKG in your 30s, which can be used for comparison with any later EKGs should it be necessary.

The test is usually performed by a technician or nurse in the office of your personal physician or cardiologist. No preparation on your part is needed. You will be taken to a quiet room and asked to undress from the waist up. The spots where electrodes (flat pieces of metal) will be placed are cleaned with an alcohol swab and then dabbed with a special jelly or paste that helps conduct electricity. Four electrodes, also called leads, are placed on your wrists and ankles and held in position with rubber straps. A fifth electrode is placed on your chest and will be moved several times during the exam. This electrode is a small metal cup with a rubber bulb on the end and is held to the skin by suction. If you are especially hairy-chested, you will be shaved at the spots where this electrode will be placed.

Once the electrodes are in place, you will be asked to remain quiet and still. The leads are connected to a machine that amplifies the minute signals generated by your heart and records them on graph paper that moves forward at a constant rate. Though it is electric, it does not send any electricity to you and there is no chance of being shocked. The standard diagnostic EKG is called a 12-lead electrocardiogram. Although 12 electrodes are not used, 12 separate tracings are made, each one using a different combination of signals from the 4-limb electrodes and the 1 chest electrode, which may be moved to as many as 6 different positions. The 12 tracings give a comprehensive view of the heart, almost a 3-dimensional portrait of its electric activity.

Many hear abnormalities including *abnormal rhythms, heart enlargement inflammation, abnormal levels of the minerals that regulate the heart's electrical conduction (potassium and calcium)* and *coronary artery disease* will cause recognizable changes in the pattern of the heart's electric activity. These can be recognized by a careful reading of the electrocardiograph tracings.

The value of the electrocardiogram can hardly be overstressed. However, an EKG is not a crystal ball. It shows what is happening to the heart, but cannot predict what will happen to it in the future. This is particularly true for patients with coronary artery disease and *angina pectoris,* its painful symptom. Unless a patient is having an attack of pain at the time, there is no guarantee that the condition will show up on an EKG taken while the patient is at rest. This shortcoming has largely been solved by the **Stress EKG,** an EKG taken when the heart's performance is measured during maximum exertion. (See **109**.)

HOLTER MONITOR. Certain *arrhythmias* (irregular heartbeats) are like the noises your car makes but stops making the moment you get it to the mechanic. They may be indeed significant, even if they do not show up during the 15 minutes you were hooked up to the EKG machine. To detect and study them, your doctor needs a 24-hour EKG. To get it, he or she will ask you to wear a Holter monitor, a portable tape recorder connected to 3 disposable electrodes that are taped to your chest. You will wear the Holter monitor on your belt for 24 hours while at the same time keeping a detailed record of your activities during the day. A continuous EKG is recorded on the magnetic tape and later analyzed by computer. An irregularity can be printed out and studied in conjunction with your diary, which may help determine what brings on the irregular heartbeats. A Holter monitor may also be used to evaluate the effectiveness of surgery or drug therapy. Results usually take at least a day.

75 ELECTROENCEPHALOGRAPHY
EEG/BRAIN WAVE TEST

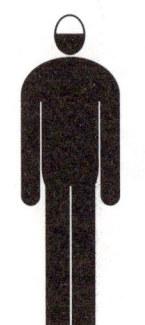

Everyone's brain gives off very small amounts of electricity, similar to, but much weaker than, the impulses generated by the heart. The patterns of these complex electrical waves can be detected by pasting electrodes (flat metal disks) to the scalp, which allow the waves to be magnified and recorded on graph paper for later study.

The printed result of this type of examination is helpful in diagnosing various illnesses and abnormalities of the brain. These conditions include *abscess, epilepsy, meningitis, tumors, blood clots, stroke* and *problems resulting from head injury.* An EEG may be able to confirm or localize an abnormality that is too subtle to be detected by x-rays or CAT scanning. However, other tests are usually needed to determine the cause of the abnormality. EEGs are also used to determine possible brain death in comatose patients.

Only your own brain impulses are measured; no electricity is administered to you. Similarly, only the pattern of your brain cells communicating with one another can be detected; this test cannot measure intelligence or *read* your mind.

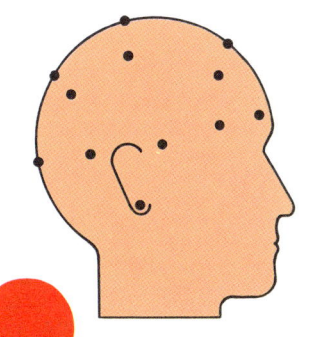

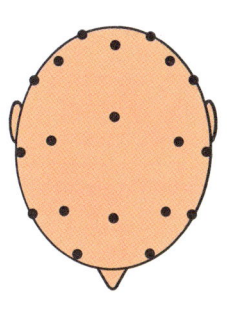

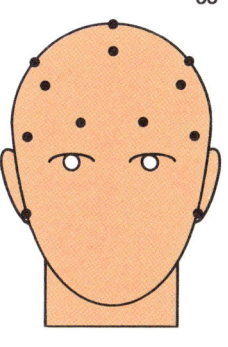

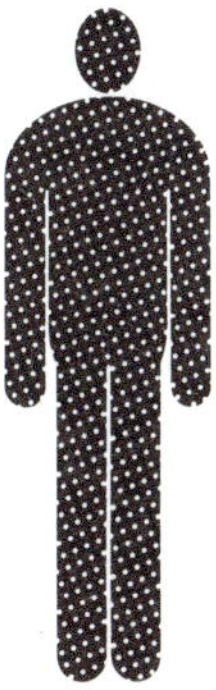

The test is performed by a technician on an outpatient or inpatient basis. The night before you are asked to shorten your sleeping time to no more than 4-5 hours. Children are permitted no more than 7 hours sleep. This deprivation of sleep helps you relax and possibly fall asleep during the study.

Your hair is not cut or shaved for the test, but you will be instructed to shampoo the night before so the electrodes can make good contact with your scalp. For the same reason, you cannot use any conditioners, oils or sprays.

You won't be asked to fast the night before the test, since hunger could produce abnormal patterns, but you will be asked to stay away from stimulants like coffee and cola and depressants like alcohol.

The test is usually performed in a special room that is shielded from outside noises. You lie on your back in a bed or a reclining chair, while the EEG technician applies 16-30 electrodes to your scalp. These are attached by means of a paste or with an elastic headcap.

Remaining still with your eyes closed, you feel nothing as the test progresses. About every 5 minutes, the recording is stopped so that you can move if you wish.

In addition to testing you while you rest, the technician may record the brain wave changes brought about by various activities. You may be asked to breathe deeply 20 times a minute for 3 minutes. A light may be flashed over your face while your eyes are open or closed, since some seizure activity is be stimulated by a flashing light.

Since some abnormal brain waves are detected only during sleep, you may be given medication to help you sleep. In this case, the EEG recordings are made while you are sleeping and waking up.

A typical EEG takes 1½-2 hours. If a sleep recording is done, the test may take 3 or more hours and afterwards you will probably feel groggy from the medication. If the sleep test is done on an outpatient basis, plan in advance to have someone drive you home.

After the test you will want to brush and wash your hair to remove the dried paste. The results of the EEG are usually interpreted by a neurologist, who reports either to you or your personal physician.

Brain death cannot be confirmed unless there are 2 *flat line* EEG recordings (recordings that show no electrical activity) taken at least 24 hours apart.

76 ELECTROLYTES

The electrolytes are 4 electrically charged minerals naturally found in the body. One of them, bicarbonate, is responsible for maintaining the body's acid-base balance. The other 3, potassium, sodium and chloride, help maintain the body's delicate fluid balance. Electrolytes are lost when there is dehydration (excessive fluid loss) due to vomiting, fever or diarrhea. This can have grave consequences on the body, in extreme circumstances leading to coma or death.

Patients taking diuretics to treat high blood pressure tend to excrete too much of the potassium electrolyte in their urine. This can lead to cramping, faintness and irregular heart rhythms; such patients may be tested regularly. In addition, because the kidney is the single most important organ involved in maintaining fluid levels, electrolytes are tested in any investigation of *kidney disease*. However, electrolyte levels can affect, and in turn be affected by, a wide range of other circumstances, so the test may be performed in cases of *diabetes, lung, heart and brain disease.*

Electrolyte testing is done on most patients entering the hospital because it provides important baseline information which can be referred to later, particularly after surgery. Surgical patients tend to have reduced electrolyte levels because of blood loss, wound drainage and in some cases because they are unable to take in liquids by mouth. These patients, in fact, any patient who is receiving fluids intravenously, will have blood electrolyte levels tested regularly to make sure the proper balance is being maintained. All the electrolytes can be tested from 1 blood sample. Urine may also be tested for electrolytes.

77 ENDOSCOPIC RETROGRADE CHOLANGIOPANCREATOGRAPHY ERCP

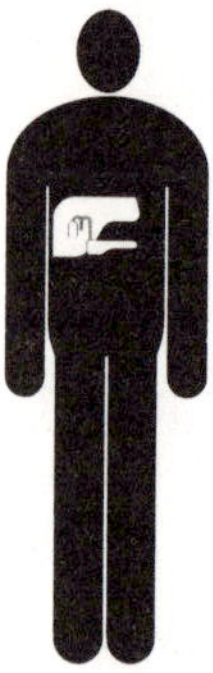

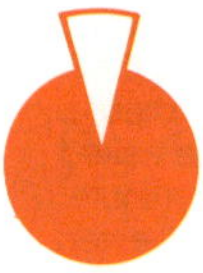

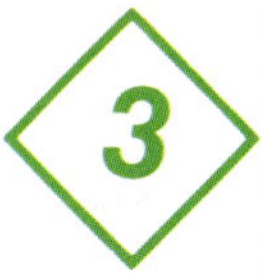

ERCP uses fiberoptic and x-ray technology to examine the bile ducts, a group of small tubes that carry bile from the liver, gallbladder and pancreas to the small intestine. The procedure is used in identifying a duct blocked by *gallstones* or *cysts*, and to differentiate between *jaundice* caused by blockage and jaundice caused by liver disease. ERCP may also help in diagnosing *cancer of the pancreas*.

The preparation for, and first part of the exam, is the same as the procedure for **Gastroscopy**. (See **81**.) You may be admitted to the hospital the day before the test and instructed not to eat or drink after midnight. Before being taken to either the radiology department or an endoscopy room, you will be sedated, probably through an intravenous line. You may also be given a drug to relax the muscles in the abdomen. As you lie on your side, the physician and an assistant guide the gastroscope into your digestive tract. The tip of the scope (about the thickness of a finger) is put in your mouth. The assistant may use his or her finger to guide the scope over the back of your tongue. You will then be asked to swallow. This is briefly uncomfortable, and you may gag, but there should be little discomfort as the physician, working very slowly, guides the scope the rest of the way down to the small intestine.

The standard gastroscope has a front viewing system, but the ERCP scope is side viewing, which makes it possible to find and manipulate the *ampulla of Vater*, a very small hole in the wall of the small intestine. Normally bile drains freely from the bile ducts into the small intestine by way of this opening. The physician may use a combination of direct viewing through the scope and moving x-ray pictures watched on a television screen to position the scope adjacent to the ampulla of Vater. Then he or she uses the scope's delicate controls to laterally extend a small hollow tube (catheter) from an opening in the scope into the ampulla of Vater. Dye is injected. As it rapidly moves through the bile ducts a series of x-rays is taken. The most unpleasant aspect of the procedure is lying very still on a hard x-ray table for up to an hour. This can be surprisingly exhausting. For several hours after the test, your blood pressure, respiration, pulse and temperature are regularly checked for signs of complication. After the anesthetic has worn off and you have full control of the swallowing mechanism you may resume a normal diet. Your throat may be sore for a day or 2.

ERCP is growing in popularity as a safe way to diagnose bile duct obstruction without resorting to exploratory surgery. In some cases, tiny forceps can be passed through the scope and into the bile ducts to retrieve stones and eliminate the need for surgery altogether.

Most patients experience no complications; however, with all procedures using dye, a patient may have an allergic reaction. Make sure you tell your doctor about all allergies you have, particularly to seafood and iodine. There is also the very remote possibility of the scope perforating the esophagus or stomach. Finally there is a risk that the injection of dye into an already blocked and infected bile duct may cause a more severe infection. To guard against this, some patients are given antibiotics 1 day before and 3 days after the procedure. The test is not recommended for pregnant or nursing mothers.

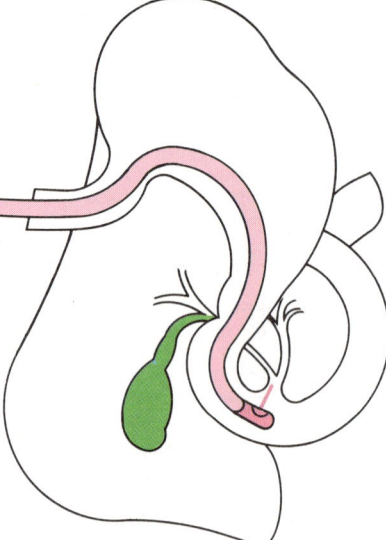

78 FETAL MONITORING NON-STRESS TEST, OXYTOCIN CHALLENGE TEST

If you have a medical or obstetric problem such as diabetes, high blood pressure, intrauterine growths, a history of stillbirth or any other problem that places your pregnancy at risk, then the health of your baby may be checked by means of an external fetal monitor which measures fetal heartrate in relation to either maternal contractions or fetal movement. It is used in several different tests done late in pregnancy and during delivery.

Two 2-inch wide rubber straps are placed around your abdomen. Attached to the straps are sensors that are positioned at different spots on the abdomen. One sensor detects the fetal heartrate using **ultrasound**. The other either senses uterine contractions or monitors fetal movement. Both relay this information to a fetal monitor, which then records it as 2 separate waveforms on the same roll of slowly-moving graph paper.

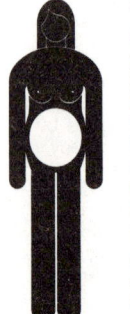

Fetal monitoring during delivery. The procedure may be somewhat uncomfortable because it requires that you remain in the same position throughout labor and cannot walk around. When labor begins, you lie comfortably on your back or side. The nurse sprinkles a small amount of talcum powder on your abdomen and positions the monitoring straps. She then applies a gel to the sensors and places them on different spots on your belly.

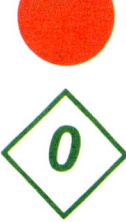

During normal uterine contractions, the flow of blood to the placenta is blocked for an instant. If the fetal heartrate (normally 120-150 beats per minute) remains steady or increases during contractions, it is a sign that the fetus is receiving sufficient oxygen and is doing well. If the fetal heartrate decreases, it could be a sign of *fetal distress,* in which the baby is not getting enough oxygen. Your doctor may then take steps to deliver the baby quickly, using forceps, vacuum extraction or cesarean section.

If everything is progressing normally during a monitoring period of 10 to 20 minutes, the fetal monitor may be removed.

Non-stress test. If yours is a high-risk pregnancy, or if your pregnancy is exceeding its predicted delivery date, this test may be performed as part of your regular obstetrical exam.

The fetal monitor is used to time the fetal heartrate simultaneously with fetal movement. A normal test, called *reactive,* will show that the baby has moved at least 2 or 3 times during a 20-minute period and that the fetal heartrate increased with each movement. If the heartrate remains the same or decreases, then the doctor will probably want to conduct more tests, such as the **oxytocin stress test,** to get a clearer picture of the situation.

Before the test begins, you will be asked to eat a meal, since a baby is more active when the mother's blood sugar level is high. After the 2 sensors are attached to your abdomen, you are asked to press a button on the fetal monitor whenever you feel the baby move or kick.

If the baby does not move for 20 minutes, then it is probably asleep, and the doctor or nurse will try to waken it by gently poking your belly or by making loud noises.

Oxytocin challenge test (oxytocin stress test). If you have already undergone a non-stress test, and your doctor has detected a problem or has received inconclusive results, then an oxytocin challenge test may be done, providing you are at least 34 weeks pregnant.

You will be given a small amount of the hormone oxytocin to induce temporary uterine contractions. A healthy baby can withstand the decreased amount of oxygen that accompanies a contraction, so if the baby's heartrate remains the same or increases during the oxytocin-induced contractions, then it will probably be fine during the natural contractions occuring at birth. However, if the test shows that the heartrate *decreases* during contractions, then the baby may not be able to withstand the rigors of an unassisted birth and the doctor may choose to perform a cesarean section. The oxytocin is usually given through a slow intravenous infusion.

If you show signs of having good contractions for 10 minutes, the oxytocin will be discontinued and the fetal monitoring will go on for another 30 minutes or so, until the contractions diminish completely, usually within an hour.

During this test, which may take as long as 2 hours, you will feel mild labor pains. Breathing exercises will help control the discomfort.

The injected hormone can induce premature labor. For this reason, the test is only performed if it has already been determined that the baby's well-being is in question.

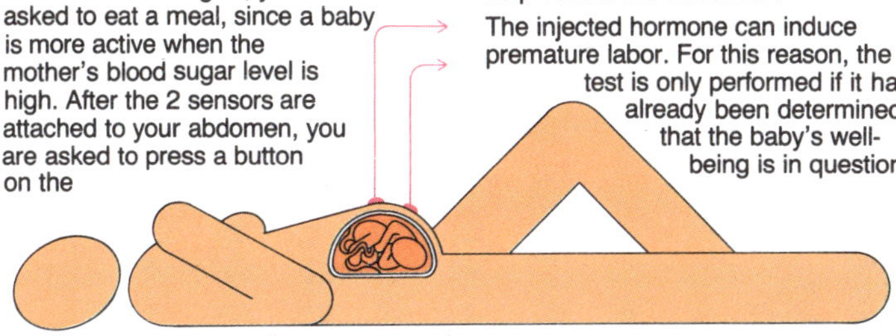

79 FUNDOSCOPY

The eye is much more than the window of the soul. When the doctor shines that bright little light and looks into your eye, he or she is looking at the

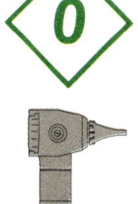

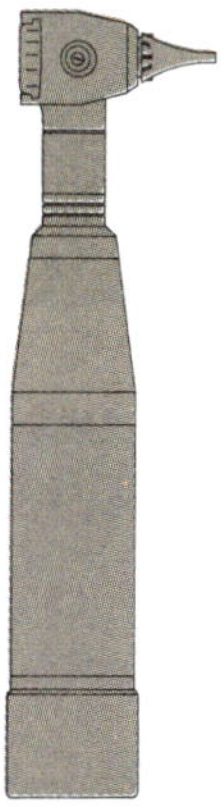

fundus, the back part of the eye which is made up of the retina, the optic disk and a network of tiny blood vessels. This is the only place in the body where veins and arteries can be directly and noninvasively observed. The procedure is an important part of every physical examination. By identifying subtle clues at the back of the eye, your physician can detect disease caused by *high blood pressure* and *arteriosclerosis,* some *brain disease* and *eye disease* caused by *diabetes,* as well as other specific ailments of the eye. Tiny blood clots may be visible in patients who have had a stroke. In a patient with *meningitis* or other disease that causes increased *fluid* pressure in the skull, the outline of the optic disk may be blurred. (The optic disk is the head of the optic nerve, which connects directly to the brain.)

The doctor doing the exam uses a fundoscope (ophthalmoscope), an instrument with a small light and adjustable lens. While you pick a point to stare at, he or she will shine the light in your eyes and look into the pupil and through the lens to the back of the eye. He or she may move the fundoscope slightly to get a better view. There is no pain associated with this examination, though some patients get nervous having the doctor so close. In some instances the doctor may want to dilate the pupil with drops. The drops sting slightly and make the eye overly sensitive to light for several hours.

Visual information travels from the optic disk to the back of the brain at a rate of 300 miles per hour.

80 GASTRIC ANALYSIS

Gastric analysis measures the amount and composition of the acidic digestive juices made by the stomach and yields important—although not definitive—information about *ulcers*. Gastric analysis is also used to detect the presence of *gastric cancer cells* and determine the effectiveness of recent ulcer therapy or surgery.

You will be asked to fast beginning midnight on the day preceding the test—no food or fluids, as these may alter the gastric secretions. No smoking either, as nicotine stimulates gastric acid secretion. The test will be administered by a nurse or a technician in a special GI (gastrointestinal) room in the hospital or in your own hospital room or doctor's office.

At the start of the test, the nurse lubricates the end of a long thin plastic tube and inserts it through one nostril, gently advancing it until you feel the tip at the back of your throat. (Occasionally, it is inserted through the mouth.) At this point, you may gag or feel an urge to vomit. If so, you may be permitted to sip some water through a straw and will probably be told to breathe deeply—either relaxes the gag reflex. In some cases, an anesthetic is swabbed on the back of the throat to help ease the passage of the tube.

You will have to dry-swallow, sip water or chew ice chips to help advance the tube down the esophagus. Once the tube has reached its final destination, the nurse tapes the tube in place at your nose. At this point, all traces of the nausea should be gone.

The contents of your stomach will be suctioned out at 15-minute intervals. After an hour, you will receive an injection of an acid-producing drug. You may feel a momentary flushing, an increase in skin temperature and itching. If the drug that is being injected is insulin (done when testing the effectiveness of recent ulcer surgery), your heart may speed up and you may feel a bit jittery and weak. More specimens will be taken from your stomach at 15-minute intervals for the next 1 or 2 hours. While the collections are being taken, you will have to spit your saliva out into a nearby basin, as saliva has a tendency to neutralize the acid content in the stomach.

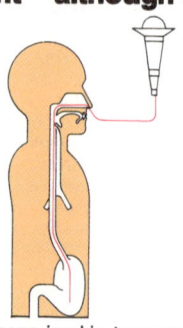

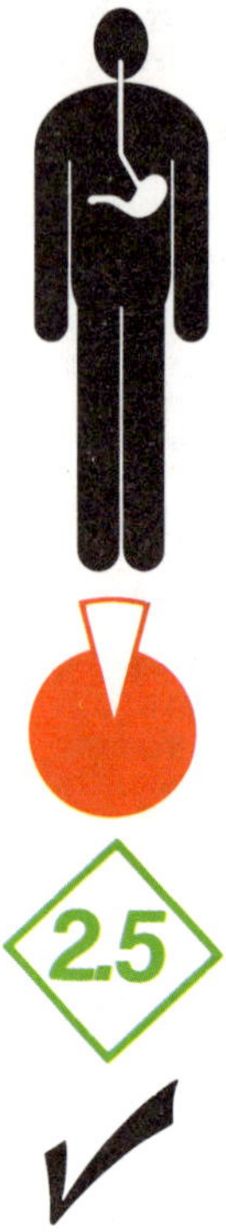

When the testing is completed, the tube will be removed—it will come out much easier than it went in. You are allowed to eat and drink again right away.

Because the test is long, anywhere from 3-5 hours, it can be exhausting, but it should only be uncomfortable while the tube is being inserted. Patients with allergies, high blood pressure or heart disease may not respond well to the injection, so be sure your doctor knows if you have any of these conditions.

81 GASTROSCOPY

Gastroscopy is a general name used for several exams similar in procedure, patient preparation and equipment. The differences among esophagoscopy, duodenoscopy and esophagogastroduodenoscopy (the tongue twister in more ways than one), have to do with how much of your gastrointestinal tract the doctors want to examine.

In all cases, a flexible fiberoptic scope called a gastroscope is used to allow a physician to directly observe the inside of the upper gastrointestinal tract which includes the esophagus, stomach and the duodenum, which is really the first part of the small intestine. The procedure may be prescribed to analyze *swallowing disorders, tumors, hiatal hernia, ulcers* and *bleeding* in the gastrointestinal tract. It is often ordered to more closely examine abnormalities that have shown up in previous x-ray studies. Gastroscopy may also be used to remove small foreign objects that have been accidentally swallowed and are lodged in the esophagus.

The test, commonly performed in an endoscopy suite of a hospital, can be performed on an inpatient or outpatient basis. Either way, you will be prohibited from eating after midnight before the test. This is not to aid in visualization, since food passes rapidly through the upper part of the gastrointestinal tract, but rather to prevent vomiting during the exam. If vomited material is inhaled, it can cause an infection or irritation in the lungs which may lead to pneumonia.

Before the test begins you are sedated. You will feel relaxed, but you will not lose consciousness. A local anesthetic is sometimes applied to the back of the throat by spraying or gargling.

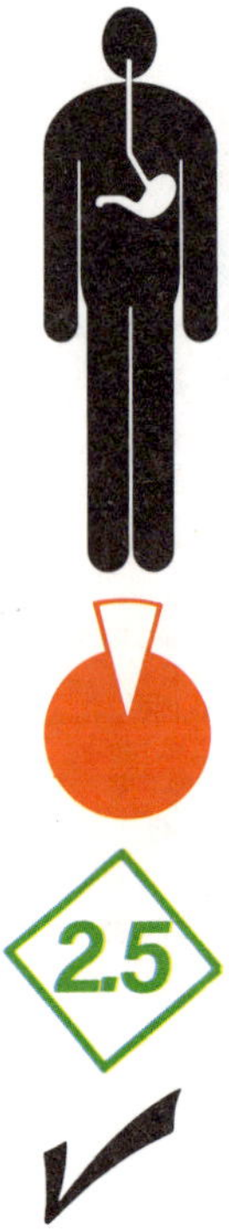

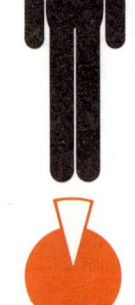

Gastroscopy can be done either lying or sitting. In either case, an assistant holds your head. The assistant or doctor places a finger in your mouth and guides the tip of the endoscope over the back of your tongue while asking you to swallow. You may gag briefly and have an urge to vomit, but this quickly passes. Once the scope is in the esophagus, a mouth guard is put in place, preventing you from biting down and ruining some very expensive equipment. The gastroscope is then slowly guided down the esophagus and into the stomach and duodenum. There may be a crampy heartburn-like feeling as the scope enters the stomach.

The main visual exam takes place after the scope has been fully inserted. It is withdrawn slowly and rotated in all directions to provide the physician with a clear view. Sites where bleeding has occurred may be washed with water forced down the scope. Tissue samples may be taken with brushes or minute forceps passed through a narrow hollow channel in the gastroscope. When the scope is finally removed, between 25 and 60 minutes later, you are asked to lower your head and cough, ensuring that no material from the gastrointestinal tract is accidentally inhaled. While not painful, the procedure is exhausting, and most patients rest for an hour or so before resuming activity. During this time, your pulse, respiration, temperature and blood pressure are monitored to detect any complications. You will not be allowed to eat for several hours, until the anesthesia wears off.

The only common aftereffect of gastroscopy is a sore throat, which will abate within a day or so. However, there are some potentially more serious complications. Some people may react poorly to the sedation, and taking tissue for biopsy may cause excessive bleeding. Rarely, the scope perforates the esophagus or stomach, a potentially dangerous condition that must be corrected by emergency surgery.

82 GONORRHEA

Gonorrhea is a sexually transmitted disease that infects approximately 3 million Americans each year. It is primarily a disease of the urinary tract, but throat, rectum, vagina and eyes may also be infected. Left untreated, it may spread to the joints, muscles, heart and brain. In women it may cause *pelvic inflammatory disease, sterility,* and *severe eye infections* in infants born to infected mothers. Fortunately, gonorrhea responds very well to antibiotics.

The symptoms in men are highly recognizable. They include frequent and painful urination and a discharge. In women, however, these symptoms, which may also include a vague abdominal pain, are often so mild that they go unnoticed. Perhaps as many as 90 percent of all women are unknowing carriers who are only diagnosed by a tracing of sexual contacts. It is critically important that all men who have gonorrhea tell all their female contacts about the exposure; otherwise the women might never know that they are infected. (Sexually active women are encouraged to have a yearly gonorrhea exam.)

There isn't a good blood test for gonorrhea yet. Instead a smear of the discharge is put on a slide, stained and examined under a microscope for direct evidence of the bacteria. This method, however, is not considered conclusive. To confirm a diagnosis the sample must be *cultured,* that is put in an environment which allows the bacteria to multiply and thereby be more easily identified. Results take between 24-48 hours. Sample taking in women follows the same basic procedure used for a **Pap smear** and is not painful. If there is no obvious discharge in a man, a Q-tip type swab may be inserted 2 centimeters into the urethra to get the sample. This smarts... a lot. Luckily it only takes a couple of seconds to do.

A fairly large dose of injected penicillin is still the treatment of choice and is quite effective. However, there are now newer strains of gonorrhea, brought over from Southeast Asia, that appear to be penicillin-resistant. cases are treated with a combination of other antibiotics.

All patients with gonorrhea should be retested after treatment. They should also be tested for syphilis which may mimic the symptoms of gonorrhea and go undetected. Though some do not comply, doctors are required by law to report all confirmed cases of gonorrhea and syphilis to a local public health authority. If you didn't give the names of recent sexual contacts to your doctor, a public employee may visit or call and request the names so that the contacts can be notified and tested. The public health employee will do the contacting for you, and without ever mentioning your name.

83 HEARING TEST *AUDIOMETRY, AUDIOGRAM*

Audiometry, the most common test for hearing loss, is simple, quick and painless. You listen through earphones to sounds produced by a machine called an *audiometer*, while a technician notes whether or not you can hear them. The audiometer is operated by a specially trained professional known as an audiologist, and the test is conducted in a soundproof room.

Sounds are sensed in 2 different ways. You hear most sounds when they are transmitted through the air *(air conduction).* A disturbance in the air produces soundwaves that are channeled through the visible part of your ear (the pinna), through the outer and middle parts of the ear, to the cochlea, a small structure in the inner part of the ear. The cochlea, shaped like a snail's shell, is filled with fluid. Tiny hairs that line the cochlea change the vibrations that reach them into nerve impulses, which are then transmitted to the brain along the auditory nerve.

Air conduction is supplemented by *bone conduction,* vibrations conducted through the bones around and behind the ear to the inner ear.

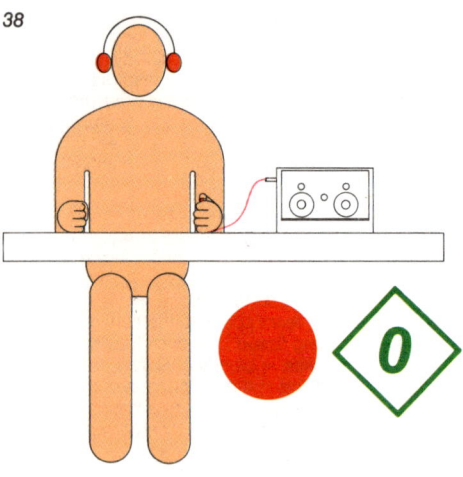

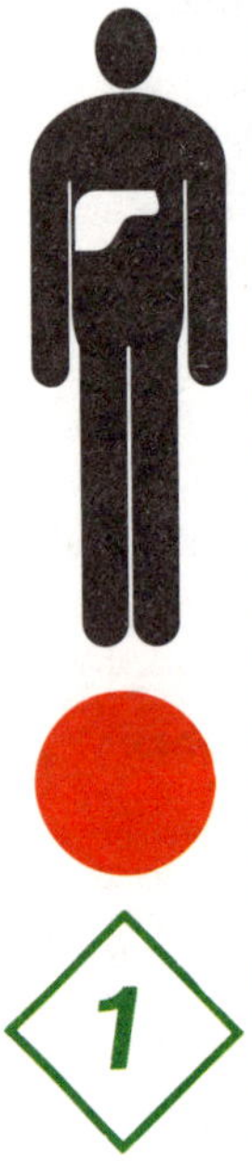

You hear your own voice mainly through this secondary kind of hearing, which is why it tends to sound differently and usually higher when you hear a tape recording.

To measure both types of hearing, the audiologist will ask you to put on a pair of earphones connected to the audiometer. You will then hear a series of tones in either one or both ears. These tones will vary in loudness and pitch (high or low). After each one has been played, you will be asked if you heard the sound and if so, in which ear. An attachment from the earphones is then placed on the bones behind the ear and the sounds are repeated.

The audiologist prepares a chart showing the lowest volume that you could hear at each pitch.

Audiometry is recommended as a standard screening test for children at age 5, before they enter school.

84 HEPATITIS

Hepatitis is a generic word meaning an inflammation of the liver. There are many possible causes of hepatitis including drugs,

alcohol and industrial toxins, but usually when someone talks about hepatitis, they are referring to hepatitis caused by a virus. There are 2 predominant types of viral hepatitis.

Hepatitis A, also called *infectious hepatitis,* is the milder disease. It is spread primarily by food, eating utensils or hands that have been contaminated with feces. (It can also be transmitted by transfusion, though this is almost unheard of.) It tends to be most common among children, young adults, and those who have traveled to high risk areas where sanitation is poor. The virus can also be transmitted through sexual contact, particularly the kind that puts male homosexuals at increased risk. Although Hepatitis A is very contagious and its symptoms—*fatigue, lack of appetite, nausea, jaundice, muscle aches*—are miserable; it is not particularly dangerous. Despite the fact that there is no medical cure, almost all patients recover completely within 3 weeks to 3 months, and there is no lasting damage to the liver.

Hepatitis B, also called *serum hepatitis,* is more severe. It is primarily spread through contact with contaminated blood by way of needles, razors, dental tools, blood products and transfusions. The virus is present in saliva, semen, nasal mucus and menstrual blood, so it can also be spread through sexual contact. Hepatitis B has the same symptoms as Hepatitis A but they tend to last longer and be more severe. Roughly 10 percent of those with Hepatitis B develop some type of chronic liver disease like *chronic active hepatitis* or *cirrhosis,* diseases that can lead to liver failure and eventually to death.

There are several blood tests designed to test for the presence of the Hepatitis A or Hepatitis B virus. Blood can also be tested for the presence of antibodies to these viruses. People suspected of having hepatitis will probably be tested several times: to establish the diagnosis, then to check on the progress of the disease and to determine whether the patient is still a carrier. In some cases, Hepatitis B sufferers who appear in good health can still carry and transmit the virus for years. Patients being tested for hepatitis may find that the personnel taking the sample take extra care not to come in direct contact with the blood which is then specially labeled and handled. Patients with hepatitis may also have **Liver Function** tests done which show how badly liver function has been impaired by the disease. These are probably more common in cases where the hepatitis is caused by alcohol abuse.

A vaccine is now available to protect against Hepatitis B, which is currently on the rise. Infection has increased 68 percent since 1978, at the rate of about 200,000 new cases a year. Doctors urge all in high risk groups to get the vaccine. Those at risk include: Homosexual men, health care professionals, prostitutes, dialysis patients, drug addicts and certain refugee groups including Haitians and Indochinese.

85 HERPES SIMPLEX II

Genital Herpes (herpes simplex II) can be diagnosed several ways. The blood can be analyzed for antibodies that fight the virus, but this is a clumsy

method requiring 2 blood tests several weeks apart. More often, a sample is taken from a lesion or sore and analyzed directly under a microscope or sent to a lab for culturing. Results are available in 2-3 days.

However, in most cases, a test is not necessary. Herpes has very definite characteristics. Simply by listening to your symptoms and visually examining a sore, most doctors can make a confident diagnosis.

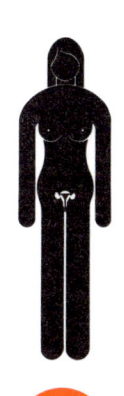

While herpes is painful and extremely contagious during attacks (when sores are present) it is not dangerous—with 1 exception. A pregnant woman who gives birth while sores are present can pass the disease on to the infant. Consequences are severe, ranging from blindness to brain damage and death. During pregnancy a definite diagnosis is critical. If active lesions are present in a woman who is near term, a cesarean delivery is performed and the danger avoided.

This does not mean that a woman with herpes can never have a vaginal delivery. However, she must work closely with her doctor to determine if her herpes infection is active. This is done by paying careful attention to the symptoms that warn her of an upcoming attack and taking periodic Pap smears and vaginal cultures. A vaginal culture is taken basically the same way as a sample for a **Pap smear**; a cotton swab is rotated around the inside of the vagina. The difference lies in how the sample is analyzed. A Pap smear sample is examined immediately under a microscope; the cultured sample is processed for several days in a lab. Culture results take longer but are more accurate. If no lesions are present in the vagina and no hidden virus has been discovered by testing, many doctors believe it is safe to go ahead with vaginal delivery.

The most obvious symptom of herpes is a sore. This usually starts as a small red spot on the penis or vagina which may be slightly raised. It turns into a small blister or cluster of blisters which burst and form small open sores. These gradually scab over and heal. There may also be other symptoms that accompany the sores. These include fever chills, swollen lymph glands in the groin, a tingling pins-and-needles sensation in the legs, itching and ache in the testicles.

Though recurrent attacks tend not to be as severe as the first attack and are less likely to be accompanied by the flu-like symptoms of fever and chills, many of the other symptoms may appear several days before the sores. You may be contagious during this period. With careful attention, you can learn to recognize these symptoms, anticipate an outbreak and stop sexual activity until it is over.

In 1985 the FDA licensed a drug called Acyclovir (trade name is Zovirax) that has had some success controlling herpes symptoms. More than 50 percent of those tested reported no outbreaks, or reported much milder and shorter outbreaks while taking the drug. The drug does not cure herpes. Once you stop taking it there is every likelihood you will continue to get outbreaks as before.

It seems safe, but until long term studies are available, doctors are being advised to prescribe Acyclovir for no longer than 6 months. Acyclovir is not for everybody; it's expensive most effective for people who have only a few mild outbreaks a year, it's probably not worth it. It is recommended for people whose outbreaks are unusually long (more than 2 weeks) or who have more than 10 to 12 severe outbreaks a year.

86 HYSTEROSALPINGOGRAM

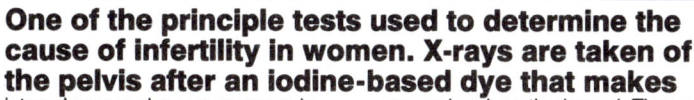

One of the principle tests used to determine the cause of infertility in women. X-rays are taken of the pelvis after an iodine-based dye that makes
internal organs show up on x-rays is inserted into the uterus and fallopian tubes. The resulting pictures will detect blocked or kinked tubes as well as any uterine abnormalities that may be hindering conception. The test may also be ordered to locate uterine tumors and to investigate persistent uterine bleeding and excessively painful menstruation. The test should be performed about 5 days after the end of your period to minimize the risk of aborting an unknown pregnancy. It should be postponed if you have any undiagnosed vaginal bleeding or any evidence of a pelvic infection.

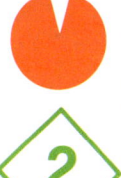

The test is usually performed in a hospital radiology department, but on an outpatient basis. The bowel must be clear for the pelvis to be visualized, so you will be given a laxative the night before the test and perhaps a suppository or enema the following morning. You may also be given a mild tranquilizer or antispasmodic pill the morning of the test.

You are instructed to urinate and are then taken to the radiology department, where a plain x-ray of the abdomen may be taken to make sure the bowel is clear. You then lie on the x-ray table with your feet in stirrups—the same position used for a conventional pelvic exam. A speculum is inserted into the vagina, the cervix exposed and gently cleaned. Then a slender tube is inserted in the cervix. You may feel a momentary spasm or transitory cramps. A moment of rest is allowed for any spasms to pass and the cervix to dilate. The dye is then injected through the tube into the uterus. X-rays are taken and more dye is inserted until the uterus and fallopian tubes are full. Insertion of the dye is uncomfortable and may feel like exceptionally strong menstrual cramps. You may be asked to change position or the table may be tilted while more x-rays are taken. The whole procedure shouldn't take more than 30 minutes.

After the test you may feel nauseous, dizzy and a bit crampy. The cramps can last for a day or 2. You should have someone with you who can drive you home. You will also have a vaginal discharge that may be bloody.

Though the test is uncomfortable, it is no more risky than any other test involving contrast material. You should, as always before such tests, tell your doctor about allergies, particularly to seafood which is high in iodine. On rare occasions, the dye has caused pelvic infection; on the other hand, the test itself has also been known to have therapeutic effects. Sometimes the passage of the dye is sufficient to clear the tubes of blockages.

87 INTRAVENOUS CHOLANGIOGRAPHY *IVC*

A lengthy, but not terribly uncomfortable study. A contrast dye is injected into a vein making the bile ducts, and to a lesser extent the gallbladder, visible on x-rays. It is most commonly performed after the gallbladder has failed to show up on an **Oral Cholecystogram**. This is often the case when gallstones or tumors are blocking the bile ducts and inflaming the gallbladder.

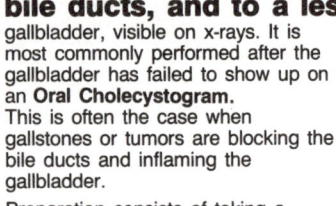

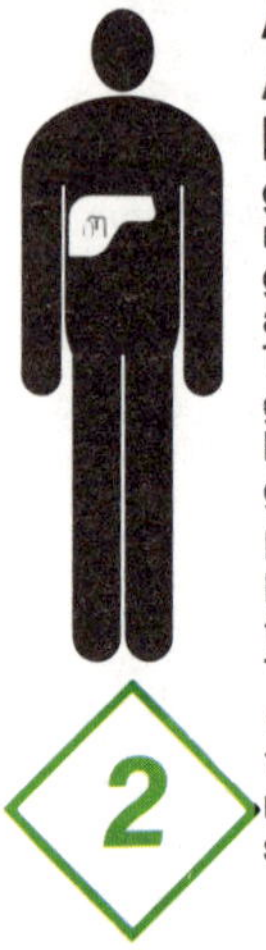

Preparation consists of taking a laxative to clear the bowel and fasting for 8-12 hours before the test. The sensation is similar to other contrast x-rays (See **Terms**). When the dye is injected, you may feel nausea and a brief flush or burning sensation. The test may take as long as 2 hours because x-rays are taken intermittently as the dye works its way through the liver, into the hepatic bile duct, and then the common bile duct. The last x-rays should show the dye entering the small intestine. Any obstructions along the way should be visible on the x-ray. You may return home after the test. Drinking extra fluids may help ease the painful urination that sometimes occurs as the dye is eliminated from the body. The test is usually not performed on pregnant or nursing mothers and patients with liver disease. Inform your doctor of any allergies you may have, particularly to iodine or shellfish.

88 INTRAVENOUS PYELOGRAPHY *PYELOGRAM, IVP*

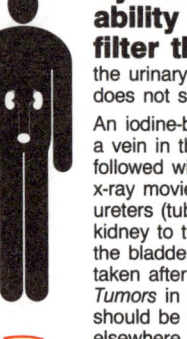

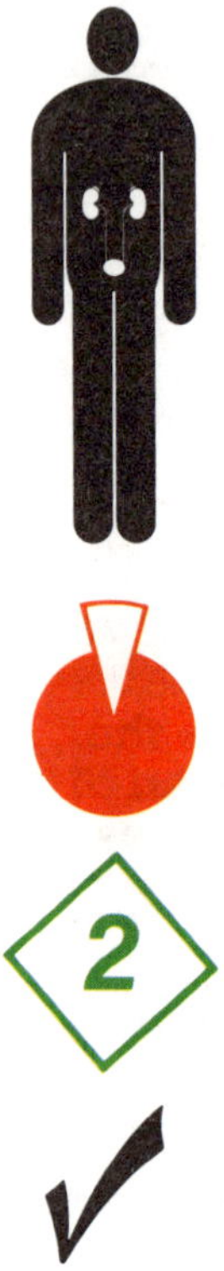

By taking advantage of the kidney's natural ability to concentrate impurities in the blood and filter them out, an IVP allows for visualization of the urinary system, which ordinarily does not show up well on x-rays.

An iodine-based dye is injected into a vein in the forearm. Its path is followed with x-rays (and sometimes x-ray movies) to the kidneys and the ureters (tubes that connect each kidney to the bladder) and finally to the bladder. Typically x-rays are taken after 5, 10, 15 and 20 minutes. *Tumors* in the kidney or bladder should be visible as well as *tumors* elsewhere in the abdomen that may be pressing on or displacing the ureters. Blockage of the ureters (perhaps due to *kidney stones*) should be apparent as well as certain abnormalities in the kidney or its blood vessels that can lead to severe *high blood pressure*.

The test is done on an inpatient or outpatient basis. Because the bowel must be empty for the doctor to see clearly, you will be given laxatives the night before the test and prohibited from eating and drinking after midnight.

Before the test gets underway, an x-ray of the abdomen may be taken to make sure the bowel is empty. As the dye is injected into a vein in the forearm, you will feel a warm flush, though some people experience this as a very uncomfortable burning sensation. The sensation shouldn't last more than a minute. You may also feel a bit nauseous and have a headache. Towards the end of the procedure you may be asked to urinate, after which more x-rays will be taken to assess the bladder's elimination capability. Moving x-rays on tape or film may be taken during urination, though this is uncommon. You should be able to resume normal activity without any problem after the test. The dye, which is an irritant, is filtered from the blood by the kidney and eliminated in the urine, so you may experience some burning upon urination. The dye can cause kidney damage in diabetics or patients who are dehydrated (more common in the elderly). This is prevented by giving intravenous fluids before the test. As with any study that requires an injection of iodine-based dye, there is a risk of allergic reaction. Inform your doctor about allergies, particularly to iodine or shellfish which is high in iodine. Also, inform your doctor if you are pregnant or think you might be.

89 LAPAROSCOPY *PELVIC ENDOSCOPY*

Though laparoscopy is considered minor surgery, it is a simple procedure, often done on an outpatient basis. Anesthesia makes it almost painless, and you are often able to resume normal activity within a day. The test requires making a small incision in the abdomen and inserting a scoping device to view the area underneath.

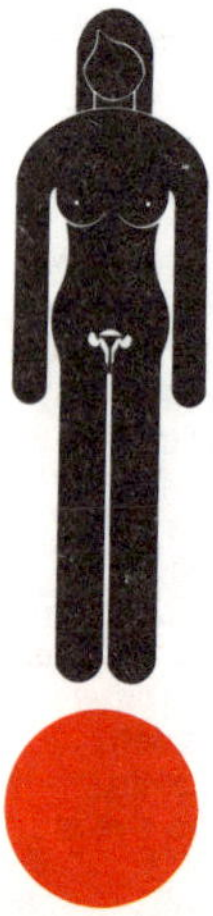

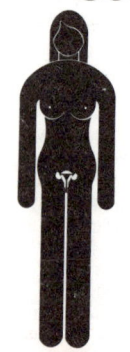

The instrument used, a *laparoscope*, is a long metal tube with a lens and tiny light source on one end and a telescopic eyepiece on the other. The scope may be used to observe the inside of the abdominal cavity and the surface of organs like the liver, gallbladder and spleen. However, laparoscopy is most frequently used to examine the female reproductive organs. The test is commonly ordered to diagnose abdominal pain or vaginal bleeding that may be caused by *pelvic inflammatory disease, adhesions* (abnormal scar tissue left from previous infection or surgery), a *uterus perforated by an IUD, cysts or endometriosis*. The laparoscope can help locate *cysts or tumors*, diagnose a *tubal pregnancy*, and investigate the cause of *infertility*. In some cases minor surgical procedures may be performed through the scope. Tissue samples may be taken for **biopsy**, adhesions or endometriosis removed, and **tubal ligation** (female sterilization) can be carried out through the scope.

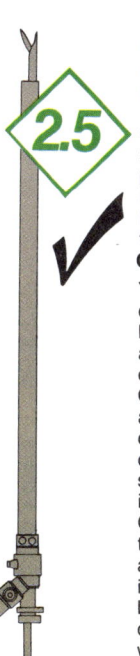

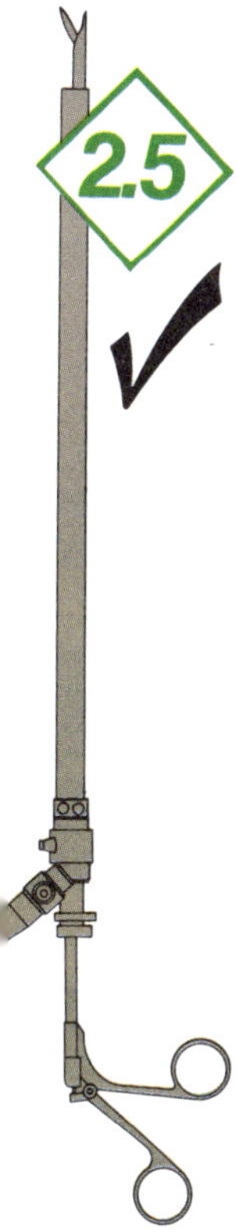

Unless therapeutic procedures are planned, where general anesthesia is preferred, the type of anesthetic used is usually something that can be decided on with your doctor. General, spinal and local anesthesia are all possibilities. If general anesthesia is used, you will probably report to the hospital or surgical clinic a day early for routine tests such as **CBC** and **Chest x-ray.**

You must begin fasting midnight the day of the test. For the test a hospital gown is worn and you go to a small operating room where you lie on a table with your legs raised. Once the anesthetic has been administered, the abdomen is cleaned and a small incision is made directly under the navel. Then a special needle is inserted through the incision into the abdominal cavity. Carbon dioxide gas is passed through the needle to inflate the abdomen. This creates a space inside the abdomen that allows for better viewing and safe manipulation of the laparoscope. The needle is withdrawn and the laparoscope inserted. The scope is angled in all directions for a full view of the pelvic and abdominal organs. If laparoscopy is used for minor surgery, another small incision may be made right above the pubic line. A second thin metal tube is inserted. Various miniature tools can be passed through the tube.

When the exam is over, both instruments are removed and most of the gas is allowed to escape. The incision(s) are closed with 1 or 2 stitches and covered with a small bandage. The whole procedure shouldn't take more than 40 minutes.

Afterwards you will rest and be watched for an hour or so for signs of complication. If there are none, you may leave the hospital. The site of the incision will be sore for a day or 2. Your abdomen may be swollen from the remaining gas, which may also cause crampy pains. You may also notice an occasional crackling sound in the skin as the gas escapes. You will probably be instructed to avoid sitdown baths for a day or 2.

Laparoscopy is considered a very safe procedure; in fact, it is one of the most common surgical procedures done in the country. However, there are rare complications that include internal bleeding, infection and perforation of the uterus, a complication that would require immediate surgical repair.

Laparoscopy has largely replaced an older procedure, **Culdoscopy,** where a scope is inserted into the pelvic cavity through an incision in the vaginal wall. Culdoscopy may still be preferred when assessing certain cancers.

90 LIPIDS   LIPID PROFILE, LIPOPROTEINS, FATS

Though there is still medical debate on the subject, it is generally accepted that there is a connection between high blood levels of lipids

(fats) like cholesterol and triglycerides and an increased risk of coronary artery disease. In order to screen for or assess this risk, blood can be analyzed in several ways. Total blood levels of cholesterol and triglycerides may be measured, but more often the blood is further broken down and analyzed for lipoproteins. These are complex molecules of fats joined to proteins. It is only in this dissolved form that fats can move freely through the body fluids and cell walls.

The lipoproteins are classified into 4 major types, 2 of which are particularly significant for heart disease. **LDL,** or *low-density lipoproteins,* seem to pick up fats in the blood and deposit them in the cells, including the cells of blood vessels, where they can develop into fatty, obstructive plugs. **HDLs** or *high-density lipoproteins,* are what the popular press commonly calls the *good cholesterol.* These molecules seem to clear the blood of excess fats and are actually associated with a decreased risk of heart attack. Therefore, while total blood fats may be important in assessing risk, the most important measure is the ratio of LDL to HDL.

Some doctors recommend testing the blood every 10 years or so, starting in young adulthood. If the levels are unhealthy, your doctor will probably recommend dietary modification and you will probably be checked more frequently. A complete breakdown can be done on 1 sample of blood. Your doctor may ask you to fast for 12 hours before the test.

91 LIVER SCAN

A nuclear scan (see TERMS) of the liver helps evaluate the organ for size, shape and function. It may be ordered to help diagnose cysts,

abesesses, tumors originating in the liver and cancer that has spread there from elsewhere. The test may also be ordered to evaluate the damage done to the liver from *hepatitis* or *cirrhosis,* or when trying to locate the best spot for a subsequent needle biopsy.

A chemical with a special affinity for the liver is labeled with very low doses of radioactivity and given to the patient by injection. Thirty minutes later, when the chemical has been absorbed by the liver, a scanning camera is passed over the abdomen. It detects the radiation and translates the absorption pattern into a picture. Except for the needle prick, the test is painless (though patients with advanced liver disease may find changing positions on the examining table uncomfortable). Radiation exposure is comparable to that received from a standard chest x-ray. This test has been largely supplanted by **CAT Scanning** which is more sensitive and capable of detecting smaller irregularities.

92 LIVER FUNCTION TESTS LFTs

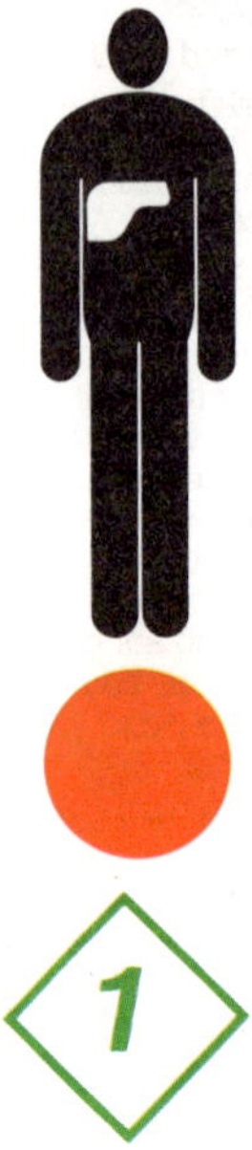

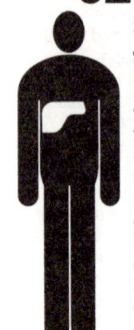

Sitting high in the right abdomen and protected by the ribs, the liver is the largest organ in the body. But unlike the heart or brain, there are no walk-through models of it in museums, no television shows dedicated to unlocking its mysteries. Few of us realize what a complex chemical processing plant the liver is. It converts glucose into material that can be stored and released later when energy is needed. It breaks down fats and also proteins, some of which it converts into the complex enzymes needed in blood clotting. It processes bile and sends it on to the gallbladder where the bile is released when fatty foods are digested. It stores vitamins, regulates hormone levels and detoxifies the drugs that we ingest as well as many poisonous waste products made by the body itself.

Some of these tests are included in **Multiple blood test panels** but the whole group is usually ordered whenever liver damage is suspected.

The tests include measurement of the blood levels of 4 enzymes and bilirubin. (See **64**.) The enzymes, *SGOT, SGPT, LDH* and *alkaline phosphatase,* are naturally produced by the liver cells either to aid in chemical processing or as by-products of it. When liver cells die because of injury or disease, these enzymes leak into the bloodstream. (Some of these enzymes are also found in the heart, brain and muscle tissue, and are released when those organs are damaged as well, but newer blood tests can isolate the tissue from which the enzymes originate.) A complete analysis of liver function might also include measuring the blood levels of certain proteins manufactured in the liver and the **Prothrombin Time** test, which measures the level of blood clotting factors made by the liver.

The 2 most common liver diseases are *hepatitis* and *cirrhosis*. In cirrhosis, chronic liver inflammation causes the organ to deteriorate. As cells die, the liver becomes shrunken, scarred and distorted. Eventually it may fail, a fatal condition. Cirrhosis may be caused by drugs, parasites, malnutrition, hepatitis and most commonly, alcohol abuse. Approximately 15 percent of all alcoholics develop some cirrhosis. Symptoms include *nausea, loss of appetite, weakness, excessive bruising* and *easy bleeding*. As the liver continues to fail, the victim may experience *jaundice, decreased sexual drive, fluid accumulation in the legs* and *abdomen, confusion, memory loss, tremors* and *varices,* distended bleeding veins in the esophagus, which constitute a medical emergency.

93 LUNG SCAN

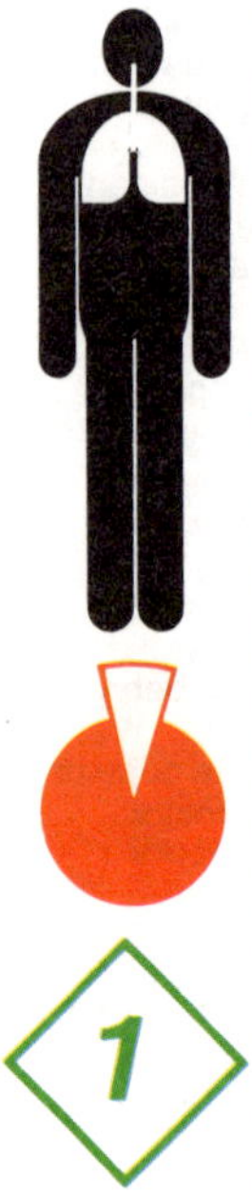

There are 2 types of lung scan. A *perfusion scan* helps determine how well the lungs are being supplied with blood. A *ventilation scan* helps determine how well air is able to move in and out of the lungs. Your doctor may order a lung scan if any of the following are suspected: *pulmonary embolism* (blood clot in the lungs), *pneumonia, asthma, bronchitis, emphysema* or *cancer.*

A perfusion scan is probably the more common of the 2 scans and is most frequently used when diagnosing pulmonary embolism. You are taken to the x-ray or nuclear medicine department where you receive an injection in a vein in your arm of a *radionuclide,* a chemical compound that has been marked with very low doses of radiation. The compound circulates in the blood; within minutes it is absorbed into the capillary structure of the lungs. While you lie on your back a scanning camera is passed over your chest. The scanner records the distribution pattern of the radionuclide in your lungs. It then translates that information into a picture your doctor can read. An area with low, uneven or nonexistent absorption of the radionuclide probably indicates an area where blood flow has been blocked by a clot. However, other disease conditions can cause a similar pattern. To confirm the diagnosis, a perfusion scan may be performed in conjunction with a ventilation scan. In a ventilation scan, a small amount of the radionuclide is mixed with oxygen, which you breathe in through a face mask. The scanning camera is passed over your chest several times: once after you first inhale the mixture, again after you have been inhaling for several minutes and finally after most of the gas has been exhaled and you are breathing plain air. You may be asked to hold your breath briefly while you are being scanned. The only discomfort associated with the test is the difficulty some people have in breathing through a face mask. *Tumors, bronchitis, pneumonia* and *emphysema* will all affect the distribution pattern of the radionuclide.

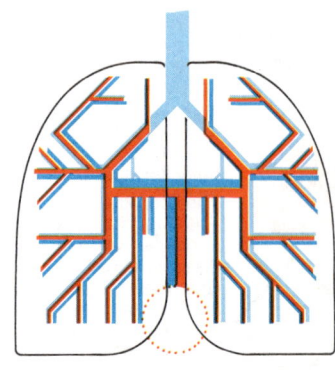

Both scans are safe and relatively painless, though patients with severely impaired lung function may find them tiring. The level of radiation exposure is roughly equivalent to what you would receive from a standard chest x-ray.

94 MAMMOGRAPHY

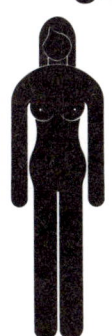

As many as 190,000 women will get breast cancer this year. If the disease is detected early, perhaps 90 percent of them will survive. Mammography is an x-ray examination of the breasts used to detect abnormalities such as *cysts, abscesses* and *tumors.* It may be ordered when a woman or her doctor has felt something unusual in the breast, when there is breast pain or nipple discharge. Though the possible implications of the exam can be psychologically distressing, and for some it is embarrassing, the test itself is quick and painless.

The exam usually takes place in a hospital radiation department. You undress from the waist up and change into a gown. The technician then helps position you according to the equipment used. Some units require you to stand, others take the x-rays while you are sitting. One breast at a time is gently placed on a photographic plate. The breast is then smoothed or compressed for better imaging with either a soft plastic shield, a sponge or a balloon device. The pressure should not be painful. Inform the technician if it is. You may be asked to hold your other breast away from the one being x-rayed. You must hold still while 2 or 3 x-rays are taken, and will probably change positions between pictures. The same procedure is repeated for the other breast. Typically you are asked to wait for a few moments while the technician or radiologist makes sure that the x-rays have come out well. The whole exam should last less than 30 minutes. While a breast x-ray can identify abnormal tissue, often a year or more before it would become identifiable by touch, it cannot positively identify it as cancerous. A final diagnosis must usually be made by **biopsy.**

Recent improvements in mammography equipment have increased accuracy while decreasing your exposure to radiation, still there is legitimate concern about all unnecessary exposure to radiation.

Every woman should examine her own breasts regularly and have her doctor examine them as part of the physical exam. Early detection is the key to surviving breast cancer and taking advantage of the less radical and disfiguring methods of treatment. Clearly for anyone who has a lump, pain or nipple discharge, the benefits of mammography far outweigh any risks. However, if you have no symptoms, history of breast disease or other risk factors, mammography is probably unwarranted as a regular screening test before you are 40. Common practice now recommends 1 baseline mammogram between 35 and 40, then every other year during the 40s, and once a year after 50, when the risk of cancer goes up.

A controversial study published in the March 1985 edition of the **New England Journal of Medicine** suggests that women with breast cancer in the early stages can be treated just as effectively by small surgery (**Lumpectomy**) and radiation therapy as by total removal of the breast, the traditional surgical treatment. Those in the study had small tumors (less than 4 centimeters or 1½ inches in diameter) with little or no spread to the lymph nodes. Their survival rate after 3-5 years was 92 percent, about the same as the rate for women who have had major surgery. As encouraging as the study is, many doctors are not satisfied with the length of time each patient was followed. Some predict that the 10-year survival rates for women who opted for the new treatment will not be as impressive. Currently, only 15 percent of all breast cancer operations are lumpectomies.

95 NUCLEAR MAGNETIC RESONANCE NMR MRI

Weighing in at 7 tons and resembling a giant insulated thermos bottle, a Nuclear Magnetic Resonance scanner is the latest advance in super sophisticated imaging technology. Like a CAT scan, it creates cross-sectional or *slice* pictures of the inside of the body, but the quality is even better. Unlike the CAT scan, NMR, or MRI (for *Magnetic Resonance Imaging*) uses no radiation or contrast dyes and can create pictures in or plane any axis.

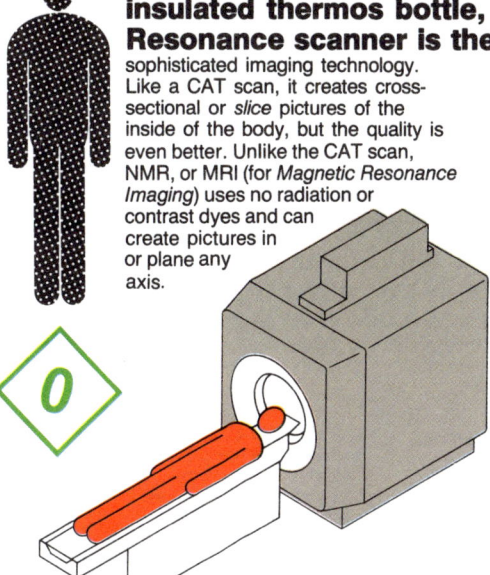

Inside the hollow of the scanner is an enormous magnet made from a 70-mile coil of niobium-titanium wire that is super cooled by a bath of liquid helium. The magnetic field generated by the scanner is powerful enough to pull a stethoscope from a physician's hands, stop watches and wipe out the magnetically encoded data on the back of a credit card. Anyone entering the scanning room must first pass through a metal detector, like those used at airports.

The word *nuclear* in NMR refers to the nucleus or center of an atom, not to radiation or nuclear power. Water molecules are the most common in the body, and each one contains a hydrogen atom. At the center of each hydrogen atom is a proton which spins back and forth generating a minute magnetic field. In the presence of the NMR scanner's much stronger magnetic field, these protons all align in one direction—the way a toy magnet will align iron filings. Once the protons are aligned, they are exposed to brief pulses of radio waves. The protons flip back and forth, absorbing and emitting the radio waves. The protons radiate the energy back at varying rates depending on tissue type and whether the tissue is healthy or diseased. These signals can be detected, amplified and then with computer enhancement, turned into amazingly detailed images. These images can help determine the most subtle clues of diseases such as *multiple sclerosis* and *Parkinson's disease* in the brain, as well as *tumors*. The technique is also being used to identify disease processes in the liver, heart and kidney. As doctors learn to interpret the images more skillfully, they hope to one day be able to spot areas likely to be affected by stroke or heart attack while there is still time for prevention.

The scanning procedure is painless; you simply lie on an examining table for several minutes while it is slid into the hollow of the cylinder. You feel nothing as the magnetic field is turned on and the radio waves are transmitted. Preliminary research shows that there is no risk from scanning. However, not everyone is a candidate for NMR. Unfortunately, anyone who has a pacemaker, metal joints or who is dependent on life-support equipment with metal parts cannot be scanned. Pregnant women are also not considered candidates for NMR scanning.

NMR, or MRI, scanners are now becoming something of a prestige item in hospitals, the CAT scanners once were, but because NMR, or MRI scanners are still in the 2 million-dollar range, they are still out of reach of all but a handful of major medical centers and research facilities.

96 OCCULT BLOOD *STOOL*

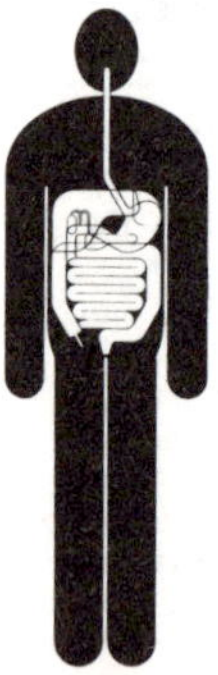

Occult blood refers to *hidden* blood that is present but not detectable by the human eye. Though urine, saliva and spinal fluid can all be chemically analyzed for occult blood, stool and urine are the substances most commonly tested.

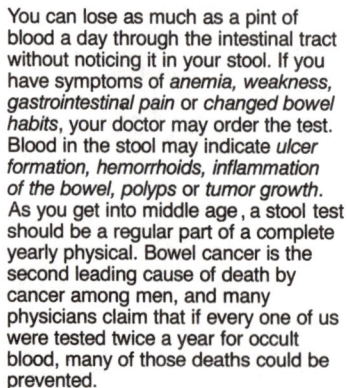

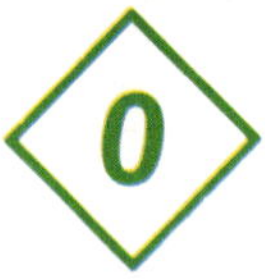

You can lose as much as a pint of blood a day through the intestinal tract without noticing it in your stool. If you have symptoms of *anemia, weakness, gastrointestinal pain* or *changed bowel habits*, your doctor may order the test. Blood in the stool may indicate *ulcer formation, hemorrhoids, inflammation of the bowel, polyps* or *tumor growth*. As you get into middle age, a stool test should be a regular part of a complete yearly physical. Bowel cancer is the second leading cause of death by cancer among men, and many physicians claim that if every one of us were tested twice a year for occult blood, many of those deaths could be prevented.

The biggest problem associated with the test is embarassment in obtaining a sample. There are several methods. If you are in the hospital or a doctor's office, you may be asked to take the sample yourself with a container and a wooden applicator. The doctor may take the sample as part of a manual rectal exam, or you may be given a *Hemoccult II* kit to take home with you. In this case you smear a stool sample on a slide or in a container and mail the kit back to your doctor for chemical analysis. Care must be taken not to contaminate the sample with urine or chemical cleaners in the toilet bowl.

A secondary problem with testing for occult blood is false positive results. False positives may result from overly vigorous teeth brushing, blood swallowed from a nose bleed or eating red meat. Turnips, aspirin, radishes, iron pills and large doses of vitamin C may also alter results, so listen carefully to your doctor's instructions. Often several samples are necessary before a doctor is satisfied with the accuracy of a positive result. If however, he or she is certain of the results, blood in the stool is strong justification for more extensive tests like **Sigmoidoscopy, Barium Enema** or a **Lower GI Series**.

Other tests done on a stool specimen include:

Analysis of fat content. Stool usually contains between 10-20 percent fat. Higher fat content could indicate *Intestinal malabsorption* or *pancreatic disease*.

Analysis for parasites and parasite eggs (ova). Sometimes called **Stool for O and P**. This is done by careful microscopic examination. Parasites that can be identified in this manner include *hookworm, amoeba, whipworm, tapeworm* and *pinworm*.

97 ORAL CHOLECYSTOGRAM *OC*

The gallbladder is a small pear-shaped sac that lies under the liver in the upper right part of your abdomen. It stores the bile that is made in the liver and releases it through a series of small tubes (bile ducts) into the small intestine, where it is used in the digestion of fatty foods.

Though the reason is not yet known, sometimes the chemicals held in solution in bile precipitate and form hard stones (not unlike the way crystals form in over-sugared water). The stones may remain in the gallbladder, often causing severe pain or inflammation when the gallbladder contracts. They may also lodge in one of the ducts causing a blockage of bile flow, which can be quite dangerous. Symptoms of gallstones include severe crampy pain in the upper right abdomen which may radiate to the front of the chest, lower back and shoulders. There may also be nausea and vomiting. Attacks of pain last anywhere from a half-hour to 4 hours and frequently follow a meal.

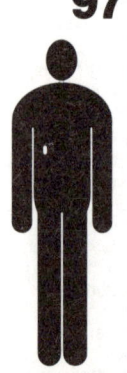

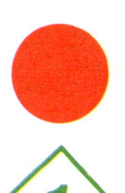

Ultrasound is becoming increasingly popular in diagnosing gallstones, but the **Oral Cholecystogram** remains the most common method. The procedure requires you to ingest pills containing iodine-based dye, which coat the gallbladder and allows it, and to a lesser degree the bile ducts, to be seen on x-rays. Whether the test is done on an inpatient or outpatient basis, the procedure is the same. The night before, you eat a low-fat dinner. Several hours later you swallow 5-6 *telepaque* pills, 1 every 5 minutes. Most patients report no ill effects from the pills, though some experience sweating, nausea, vomiting or diarrhea. Inform your doctor if this happens.

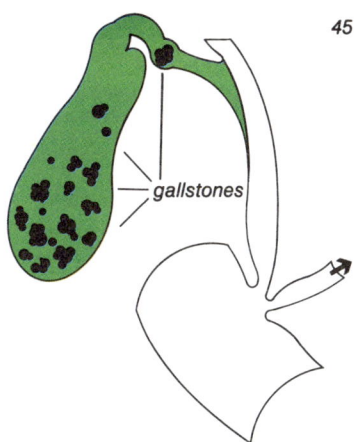

The next morning, several x-rays of your abdomen will be taken in the radiology department; the gallbladder and any stones should be clearly visible. You may be given breakfast or a fatty drink which makes the gallbladder contract and excrete more dye. In cases where the gallbladder doesn't show up, the test is repeated the next day with a higher dose of dye. If the gallbladder still doesn't show up, it's an almost certain indication of either severe inflammation or blockage of the cystic duct by a gallstone.

This is a safe, minimally uncomfortable test that shouldn't take longer than 30 minutes. The only risk is an allergic reaction to the contrast material. It's vitally important to inform your doctor of any allergies, particularly to iodine and seafood. Also tell your doctor if you are pregnant or may be pregnant.

Fair, fat, female, 4 and 40 is a rather tasteless old aphorism used to describe those most at risk for gallstones—overweight women, who are 40 or over and who have had more than 3 children. Although it is a bit simplistic, women are far more likely to get gallstones than men are, particularly women who have been pregnant. People over 60 and people who eat a great deal of animal fat and dairy products are also at risk.

98 PAP SMEAR CERVICAL SMEAR, CERVICAL SCRAPE, PAPANICOLAOU TEST

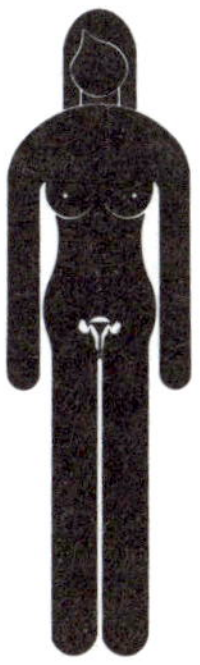

A Pap smear is almost always part of a complete gynecological examination. The test is 90-95 percent successful in detecting cancerous and pre-cancerous cells of the cervix. More importantly, the test detects the condition years before other symptoms appear. Although the incidence of *cervical cancer* is high, the cure rate, with early detection, is likewise high.

When the test was invented by Dr. Papanicolaou in 1928, cervical cancer was almost always fatal, largely because of late detection. Since the 1950s, the test has become routine, and death from cervical cancer has decreased by half. Physicians maintain that if every woman had a yearly Pap Test, death from cervical cancer could be eliminated entirely. Presently, 40 percent of American women are tested on a regular basis. A Pap Test may also be used to study suspected hormone imbalance and to diagnose viral infections of the urogenital and reproductive systems.

Since the test is dependent on a sampling of cells normally shed by the body, you are advised not to douche or have intercourse for 24 hours before the test, and to reschedule the appointment if you're menstruating. Semen and menstrual blood make it impossible to analyse cervical cells.

The physician or nurse practitioner inserts a speculum in the vagina. (It should be dipped in warm water first for your comfort, and you shouldn't feel bad about reminding them.) The speculum holds back the vaginal walls and allows the doctor to examine the cervix, the neck of the uterus and to take samples.

Typically 3 samples are taken. One is taken with a long cotton applicator Q-tip just inside the cervix. Another, also with a long q-tip, is taken from the vaginal pool—the bottom of the vagina just before the cervix. A third is taken with a wooden spatula which is scraped around the opening of the cervix with a firm circular motion. The whole procedure takes less than 5 minutes. Some find the position embarassing and the sample-taking a bit uncomfortable, but it isn't considered painful. While you are still in the room, the cell samples are smeared on slides which are then sprayed with a fixative before going to a lab for *culturing* and microscopic examination. Lab results are available within 48 to 72 hours. (A culture for gonorrhea is frequently done at the same time.)

Pap smear results are classified I-V by degrees of abnormality observed by a pathologist (I is considered normal). False positive results are possible and mild abnormalities can be caused by vaginal infection, herpes or other causes, and will disappear when the infection clears. Mild abnormalities are usually retested the following month.

Colposcopy (See **69**) is usually indicated after a series of abnormal Pap smears.

Since a connection between genital herpes and a slightly higher incidence of cervical cancer has now been established, many doctors recommend that their patients with herpes have a Pap Test twice a year instead of once every 1 or 2 years as is recommended for most women. Some doctors recommend that women taking the pill also be tested biannually. Also, women whose mothers took DES *(diethylsilbestrol)* during the 50s and early 60s may need more frequent Pap smears

Results of a Pap Test may be classified as follows:

Class I: All clear. No atypical or abnormal cells.

Class II: Atypical cells but no evidence of cancer. (Minimal cause for worry, frequently caused by inflammation of the cervix.) Another Pap Test is usually ordered 1 to 3 months later.

Class III: Findings suggestive but not conclusive for premalignant cells. (More evaluation needed, another Pap test, Colposcopy, perhaps a biopsy

Class IV: Abnormal cells strongly suggestive of cancer. (A biopsy is usually performed.)

Class V: Cells conclusive for cancer. (Requires treatment.)

The typical yearly gynecological examination includes a check on height, weight, blood pressure, examinations of the abdomen and breasts, a Pap test, **urine analysis, CBC** and a pelvic and rectal examination.

99 POSITRON EMISSION TRANSAXIAL TOMOGRAPHY *PETT SCAN*

A state of the art development in nuclear medicine, Positron Emission Transaxial Tomography or PETT scanning, provides a window into the brain.

It combines elements of CAT scanning and Nuclear scanning (See **Terms**), but the result is more accurate and informative than either. PETT traces the distribution pattern of special radioactive isotopes that are injected into the body, and then, using the same sort of computerized image enhancing technology that is used on spy satellites, translates the information into color pictures of the inside of the brain.

The total unit consists of a huge hollow cylinder and a *cyclotron*, a 5-foot cube that weighs about 25 tons. The cyclotron is used to manufacture the delicate isotopes, low level radioactive chemicals. (Some of these compounds are so fragile that they will deteriorate beyond the point of usefulness if they're not used within 2 minutes.) The isotope is combined with an organic chemical and then injected into a vein while you lie on an examining table with your head inside the hollow of the cylinder. The isotope travels to the brain where the radiation distribution pattern is recorded from multiple angles and assembled by computer into a single image or series of images.

What makes PETT so different from conventional nuclear scans is the type of chemical that can be labeled and traced. Chemicals like glucose, certain fatty acids and neurotransmitters (chemicals involved in thought transmission) are able to cross the blood brain barrier and thus reveal not only basic anatomy but also what is happening inside the brain on a chemical or metabolic level. Normal and abnormal tissue absorb the isotope and emit the radiation differently, allowing tremendously subtle distinctions to be made. *Tumors* can be identified, as can the parts of the brain responsible for *epileptic seizures,* and a variety of other mental illnesses. Shifts in blood distribution help doctors identify areas that have been affected by a stroke or blood clot and one day may help doctors locate areas that are at risk before a stroke happens.

By revealing the metabolic processes and the shifts in blood flow that accompany various types of mental activity, researchers are also using PETT to *map* the brain. They are actually able to determine what areas *light up* during activities like reading, counting and remembering. In fact, the PETT is so sensitive that patients being scanned must have their eyes and ears covered to limit extraneous sensory stimulation that could affect scanning results.

Other than the pain of an injection, scanning is painless, and preliminary studies show it to be as safe or safer than conventional x-rays and nuclear scans. On the down side, PETT scanning offers so much information that scientists are still learning how to interpret it and recognize what a normal brain should look like. Also, the technology is still very expensive (about 2.5 million dollars for scanner and cyclotron) and currently available in only a few major medical centers.

100 PLETHYSMOGRAPHY VENOUS AND ARTERIAL IMPEDENCE PLETHYSMOGRAPHY

This is a painless, noninvasive way to detect a *thrombus*—a clot attached to the wall of a vein—usually in the leg. While it is not as conclusive as **Venography**, an invasive procedure, Plethysmography is gaining in acceptance as a screening test for those at risk and where weak veins or a low pain threshold prevents injecting x-ray contrast dye.

The test is done in your room or in a hospital's vascular studies lab. You lie on your back while an occlusion cuff is wrapped around your thigh, just like the cuff used in taking blood pressure, only larger. Smaller cuffs are placed around the calf and the ankle. Wires are connected from the various cuffs to a *Pulse Volume Recorder* or *Plethysmograph* (a machine that measures the volume of blood within the leg). The volume of the leg at rest is recorded. Then the cuffs are inflated, constricting the flow of blood in the leg. This volume is also recorded, after which the cuffs are quickly deflated. The plethysmograph continues to measure the flow of blood rushing out of the area. With measurements taken at 3 different points, differences in blood flow (between thigh and calf and calf and ankle) will help your doctor pinpoint the location of any blood clot or narrowed vessels. First one leg is tested, then the other. You may be asked to raise and lower the leg. Both veins and arteries may be tested.

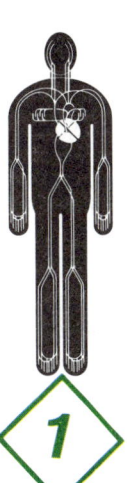

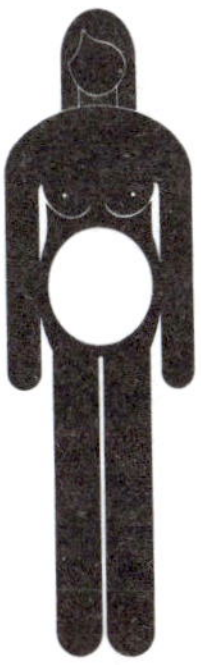

The importance of this test is detecting a deep venous clot that could possibly detach and travel to the lung. The test is commonly performed when the risk of *thrombosis* is high: after surgery that has kept the patient on the operating table for a long time, when a patient has been confined to bed, after pregnancy and when there is undiagnosed swelling in the legs. The test may be performed in conjunction with **Doppler Ultrasound.** (See 72.)

101 PREGNANCY

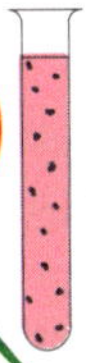

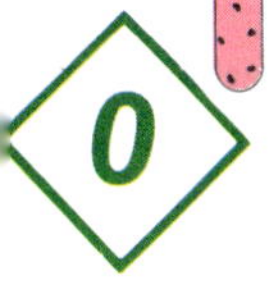

When the fertilized egg moves into the uterus and attaches itself to the uterine wall, tissue forms which will eventually become the

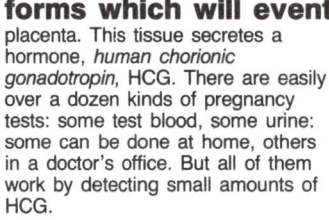

placenta. This tissue secretes a hormone, *human chorionic gonadotropin,* HCG. There are easily over a dozen kinds of pregnancy tests: some test blood, some urine: some can be done at home, others in a doctor's office. But all of them work by detecting small amounts of HCG.

Most of the tests depend on agglutination, which can be observed directly. Your urine or blood is mixed with a chemical preparation on a slide or in a test tube. If HCG is present, particles clump together in the sample. If HCG is not present, the particles will remain dispersed.

In general, urine slide tests, which only take 90 seconds, are less accurate than urine tube tests, which take 2 hours to work. Urine tests are about 80 percent accurate if performed at least 10 days after the first missed period. In order to get the best results, the first morning specimen of urine is used, where HCG concentration will be highest. When using home kits, read the package carefully. Certain drugs like penicillin and many tranquilizers alter results.

Blood can also be tested for HCG. The results are practically 100 percent accurate and pregnancy can be detected 2-3 days after conception. However, the test is more expensive, and the sample must be analyzed by a lab.

The standard symptoms that might suggest pregnancy are: *missed menstrual period; sensitive, swollen breasts; frequent urination; nausea; change in appetite; fatigue.*

The following is a list of tests commonly performed during pregnancy.

Complete blood count (CBC)	Pap smear
Rubella titer (German measles)	Glucose
	Urinalysis
Syphilis test	Blood type and Coombs' test
Gonorrhea culture	

102 PULMONARY FUNCTION TESTS LUNG FUNCTION PFTs

There are a number of noninvasive tests designed to evaluate breathing ability and the efficiency of the oxygen/carbon dioxide exchange that takes

place in the lungs. Some are quite complicated and involve breathing into measuring machinery for long periods of time, inhaling harmless gases like helium or breathing while in special chambers that regulate atmospheric pressure. However, the tests you are most likely to encounter are the simple lung or pulmonary function tests (PFTs). These can be performed at bedside, in your doctor's office or in the pulmonary function lab of a hospital. They all involve a *spirometer,* a machine that measures the rate and volume of your breath as you breathe into a hollow tube attached to it. The measurements are recorded on moving graph paper and are read very much the way an electrocardiogram is read. Your results are compared to a list of *normal readings* grouped by age, sex, weight and height.

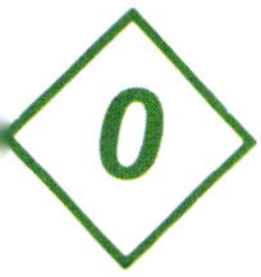

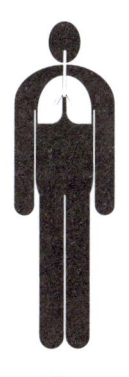

Many measurements can be taken. These are 4 of the most common:

Forced Vital Capacity. Measures how much air you can forcefully exhale after breathing in as deeply as possible.

Forced Expiratory Volume. Measures how much air is exhaled during the first second of exhalation. (An important test because patients with obstructive lung diseases like *asthma* or *emphysema* may actually exhale an almost normal amount of air. However, initial airflow may be decreased by obstructed airways.)

Maximal Mid-expiratory Flow. Measures the rate of air flow during exhalation.

Maximal Voluntary Ventilation. Measures the total amount of air you can inhale and exhale in 1 minute.

The procedure for these tests is basically the same; in fact, the first 3 can be recorded at once. You simply place your mouth around the cardboard or plastic mouthpiece at the end of a flexible tube attached to the spirometer. Then breathe as directed. You may be asked to wear noseplugs or hold your nose. During Maximal Voluntary Ventilation you will only be asked to breathe hard for 15 seconds. The result is multiplied by 4.

Except for people with severely diseased lungs, these tests shouldn't be painful or tiring. The whole procedure takes 10-30 minutes, depending on how many times you are asked to repeat the functions. In some instances the tests may be done while you breathe oxygen through a face mask. Asthmatics may have the test performed before they are given drugs which dilate the airways. Then the tests will be done again to monitor the effectiveness of treatment. An **Arterial Blood Gas** test is commonly performed in conjunction with pulmonary function tests.

PFTs can help diagnose and monitor *pneumonia, emphysema, asthma, chronic bronchitis,* and in some cases a *tumor in the lung*. Your doctor might order them if you present any of the following symptoms: *wheezing, shortness of breath, coughing, difficulty breathing* or *tightness in the chest*. The tests may be included in a complete physical for people who smoke heavily or who are exposed to hazardous fumes and dust at the workplace. They are also commonly performed before and after surgery, particularly chest surgery, and especially in older or obese patients.

103 PULSE

Your pulse rate is the number of times your heart beats per minute. Each time the heart contracts, it sends a wave of blood through the arteries. You

can feel the force of the wave yourself at the inside of the wrist just below the base of the thumb and on the side of the neck just underneath the jawline. Each of us has a resting pulse rate of somewhere between 60-80 beats per minute.

Pulse is always checked during a standard physical exam. Weak or irregular pulse beats may indicate heart or circulatory disease. Pulse can also be detected on the sides of the ankles, behind the knees and inside the crook of the arm. All these points may be checked on both sides of the body during a complete physical. The examiner mentally compares the intensity of the pulse on both sides of the body to help determine circulatory blockages.

Pulse, along with respiratory rate, blood pressure and temperature, is one of the 4 *vital signs* that are checked frequently after an invasive test or surgery.

104 RADIOACTIVE IODINE UPTAKE (RAI) AND THYROID SCAN

The concept behind both of these tests is essentially the same. Your thyroid gland, a small butterfly-shaped gland at the base of the neck,

uses iodine—present in small quantities in the food you eat—to manufacture the thyroid hormones that regulate the rate of metabolism. When more thyroid hormone is being produced, more iodine is collected from the bloodstream. If iodine is labeled with low levels of radioactivity and injected into the bloodstream, the thyroid gland's reaction to it can be measured and its function assessed.

The Radioactive Iodine Uptake (RAI) test, which can be done either in a hospital radiology department or in a laboratory, is almost always done on an outpatient basis. Typically, you report to the testing location in the morning (you may be asked to fast or eat only a light breakfast first), where you are given several pills containing a radioactive iodine compound. You are then asked to return to the laboratory anywhere between 2 and 24 hours (usually 24) later for scanning.

During scanning you lie on your back on an examining table with your head stretched back. A machine that may be called a *counter, gamma camera* or *scintillation scanner* is held over your neck. Like a Geiger counter, it does not emit radiation but very accurately measures the amount of radiation in you. In other words, it measures the ability of your thyroid to collect and concentrate iodine. You may be scanned again several hours later. Scanning is painless and usually takes less than 30 minutes.

Thyroid scanning, which is often done at the same time as RAI, goes one step further. A different kind of scanning equipment reads the radioactive iodine distribution pattern and turns it into a picture. The picture helps indicate the size of the gland, as well as areas of abnormally high or low absorption which might indicate *cysts, nodules* or *cancerous tumors.*

In general, these tests are performed only after blood tests have indicated that there is some kind of thyroid malfunction. However, the scan may also be ordered after a physical examination in which your doctor has felt a lump or nodule in the thyroid gland. These nodules are fairly common and over 85 percent of them turn out to be benign. Thyroid scans are also used to help precisely locate a nodule for needle biopsy, the only sure way to determine if the lump is cancerous.

While these tests are considered safe, the iodine compound can be harmful to someone who is allergic to iodine or seafood, which is very high in iodine. Make sure you inform your doctor if this is the case. The test is also not usually performed on anyone currently taking thyroid medication or on anyone who has had a contrast dye x-ray study performed within several months.

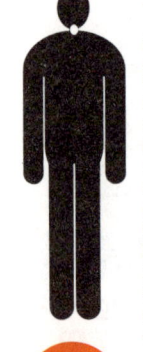

Goiter, a swelling in the neck caused by an enlarged thyroid gland, is frequently the result of iodine deficiency. This type of goiter is typical in areas where the soil and water are iodine free. At one point, at least 10 percent of the population of Ohio, Minnesota, the Great Lakes Region and the Pacific Northwest, had visible signs of goiter, but this has been largely eliminated by the widespread use of iodized salt.

105 RENAL ANGIOGRAPHY

Renal angiography is a study of the arteries that supply the kidneys with blood. However, because arteries and internal organs like kidneys don't show up well on x-rays, an x-ray resistant dye is injected into the blood to outline them clearly and allow identification of any abnormality. In renal angiography, a thin plastic tube (catheter) is placed in the *femoral artery,* a large artery in the groin, and carefully manipulated until it is close to the kidney. Dye is injected through the catheter. It enters the kidney arteries directly and a series of x-rays is taken. The large and small blood vessels of the kidney should be clearly visible. The procedure may be ordered to diagnose *tumors of the kidney* and *narrowing of the kidney arteries,* a condition that causes severe high blood pressure and requires surgical repair.

Though the test can be done on an inpatient or outpatient basis, you may have many of the standard pre-surgery tests performed, including **blot clotting studies** and **blood typing.** You will be instructed not to eat or drink after midnight. The next morning you will be taken to an angiography room, which may be a small surgical suite or a separate room in the radiology department. While you lie on an x-ray table your groin is draped with sterile cloth and cleansed. The skin is numbed with an injection of local anesthetic. This stings briefly. When the skin is numb, the doctor makes a small incision to expose the femoral artery. The artery is pierced with a needle. A thin guide wire is passed through the needle and the catheter is slipped over the guide wire as the needle is withdrawn. Above you, a fluoroscope takes moving x-ray pictures. Your doctor watches these on a tv set and uses the information as he or she guides the catheter into position. Reaction to catheter insertion varies widely among patients. Some feel only an unusual pressure while others are extremely uncomfortable. It is important to remain very still during this part of the procedure, which doesn't make it any easier.

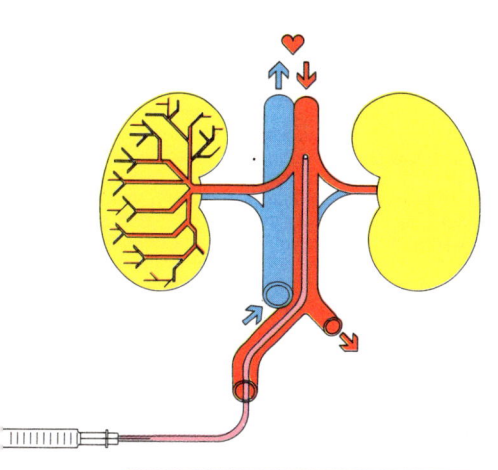

Once the catheter is in position, the dye is injected and several x-rays taken in rapid succession. When the dye is injected, you will feel an intense burning sensation and perhaps some nausea. This should pass quickly. If it does not, inform your doctor. A few minutes later, when the dye has moved from the arteries to the veins, more x-rays may be taken.

After the catheter is withdrawn, direct pressure is applied to the puncture site in the groin for 5-15 minutes and then a pressure dressing is applied. You will be instructed to rest in bed for several hours while the incision is watched for swelling and bleeding. Cold packs may be applied to the puncture site. Your pulse, blood pressure, temperature and leg pulse will be checked frequently for signs of complication. You will be encouraged to drink fluids to reduce dehydration, a common aftereffect of the dye. Hospital bedrest is usually ordered for a day while the incision heals.

There is a small degree of risk associated with this procedure. Allergic reaction to the dye is a rare but possible complication as is excessive bleeding. It is also possible that the catheter insertion and dye infusion could dislodge a blood clot or a fatty plaque in an artery. This could travel to another smaller blood vessel, perhaps blocking the flow of blood to the legs or an internal organ. As with all x-rays requiring dye injection, you must tell your doctor about all allergies, particularly to shellfish or iodine. This test is not usually performed on pregnant or nursing mothers.

106 SEMEN ANALYSIS *SPERM COUNT*

Infertility affects approximately 10 percent of married couples in America. A doctor will generally decide to investigate infertility after a couple has tried unsuccessfully to conceive for a full year during which no contraceptives have been used. If there has been no conception during the year, a Semen Analysis, which is inexpensive, painless and non-invasive, is often the first test ordered in a full fertility workup.

For the analysis, the lab requires a sample of the man's semen in a clean glass container within an hour of ejaculation. (After a longer period of time, the sample deteriorates.) To obtain the freshest sample, the man will be asked to masturbate in a private place, either in the doctor's office or the lab. Less desirable, but sometimes necessary due to extreme embarrassment or religious conviction, is sample collecting after withdrawal (coitus interruptus). If you collect the sample at home, be sure to use a sterile container (usually one will be provided). You must, however, get it to the lab promptly, without letting it get too hot or too cold. Because frequent sexual activity reduces both the volume of the sample and the number of individual sperm in it, you will be asked to refrain from intercourse for 3-5 days before the test. You may also be told to avoid drinking alcohol, which has an adverse effect on sperm number.

In the lab, the sample is analyzed for volume, viscosity (thickness), number of sperm, cell structure and mobility, the ability of the sperm to move or *swim* up the vaginal canal to the fallopian tubes where fertilization takes place. At least 2 and sometimes 3 samples must be taken months apart before infertility can be confirmed.

A normal sperm count is anywhere between 20 and 60 million sperm cells per milliliter of semen. Anything less and the chances of conception are statistically reduced, though conception is not precluded. Fatigue, stress, excessive alcohol or tobacco ingestion, as well as heat effects on the scrotum from binding underwear, may all lower the sperm count. Other causes of infertility in men include *mumps,* particularly mumps in adulthood, *hormone deficiencies* and *variocele,* a defect in the testicular vein. Roughly half of all infertile males can be treated successfully with either a change in lifestyle, hormone therapy or by surgery.

107 SIGMOIDOSCOPY *PROCTOSIGMOIDOSCOPY*

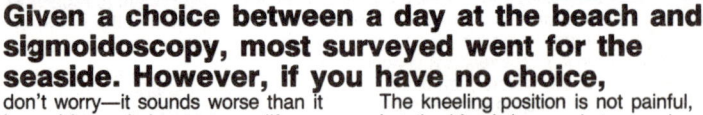

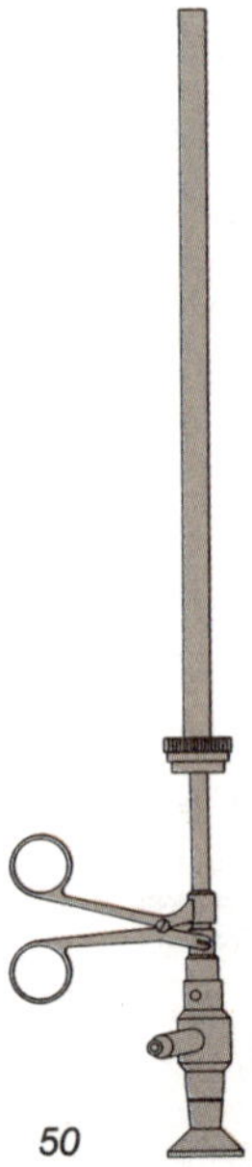

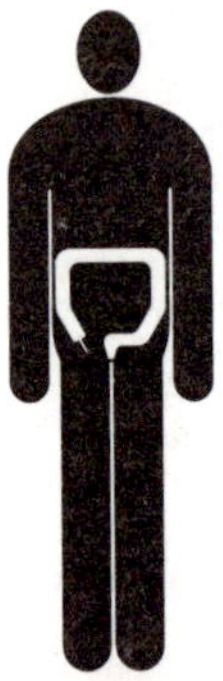

Given a choice between a day at the beach and sigmoidoscopy, most surveyed went for the seaside. However, if you have no choice, don't worry—it sounds worse than it is, and it can help save your life.

In brief, sigmoidoscopy is a procedure that allows the physician to examine the lower 10-12 inches of the large intestine and rectum. He or she uses a *sigmoidoscope* (a *proctoscope* is shorter and is used if only the rectum is being examined) which is a flexible or rigid tube about a foot long and as thick as a cigar. It has a light source, a magnifying eyepiece and an open channel through which air can be passed and biopsy samples taken.

It is an important procedure because *cancer of the bowel* is the second largest cause of cancer deaths among men, and 65 percent of such cancers are within identifying reach of the physician's finger or the sigmoidoscope. The test is also used in diagnosing diseases of the bowel such as *diverticulosis, polyps* and *ulcerative colitis.* It is likely to be prescribed if you are experiencing rectal pain, a radical change in bowel habits, or especially blood in the stool. (If you are a man over 45 with a family history of bowel cancer, the test may be ordered regularly as part of a full physical.)

The procedure is performed by a family physician, internist or gastroenterologist and may be done on an inpatient or outpatient basis, in your hospital room or in a doctor's office. Whether you'll receive an enema and/or laxative beforehand depends on your physician. Some maintain a cleansed bowel facilitates viewing, while others feel that enemas alter the mucosal lining of the bowel and interfere with diagnosis. Though you may request it, typically no sedation or anesthesia is needed or given.

Sigmoidoscopy is usually performed in a kneeling position with your head down and buttocks raised. Some doctors have special examining tables that are designed for this position. It may also be performed as you lie on your left side with a sandbag under your hip to raise it. The kneeling position is not painful, but the blood does rush to your head and many feel extremely vulnerable and embarrassed. To help ease the feeling of exposure, you will be draped with sheets or allowed to wear a gown.

Before inserting the scope, the physician examines the exterior of the anus and performs a manual exam of the rectum. A gloved and well lubricated finger is eased into the anus. The doctor should be able to feel muscle weakness, fissures and irregularities or masses that may be pressing on the passageway from outside the rectum.

The finger is removed and the scope slowly inserted. Air may be forced through the scope to expand the bowel, making insertion and visualization easier. The air may make you feel crampy or like you have gas pains. Insertion of the scope itself is an uncomfortable, bizarre feeling. You may have a strong urge to defecate, but it isn't really painful. If you find yourself involuntarily tightening, breathing deeply through the mouth should help you relax. The physician will have had his eye to the eyepiece for most of the insertion and he will continue to observe closely while the scope is rotated slowly and withdrawn. If he has seen polyps or suspicious tissue, a tiny forceps may be passed through the scope and a tissue sample (*biopsy*) taken. This is painless.

The whole procedure should last 15-20 minutes and once the scope is withdrawn, cramps and the feeling of fullness disappear. You may, however, feel a bit woozy and want to rest on the table before getting up. If you think you need help, ask for it. In some cases your physician can report on his or her observations immediately. If tissue samples have been taken the full report takes 2-4 days. You should be able to resume normal diet and activities immediately. A slight bit of blood in the stool following sigmoidoscopy is normal, particularly if there has been a biopsy. If the bleeding seems heavy or persists, report immediately to your physician.

Sigmoidoscopy is considered a safe procedure; nevertheless, there are risks. Rare complications include perforation of the bowel and heavy bleeding upon removal of a polyp or tissue sample. These risks should be discussed with your physician.

108 SPINAL TAP CEREBROSPINAL FLUID TEST

Cerebrospinal fluid (CSF) is a clear fluid produced in the brain. It surrounds the brain and flows down and around the spinal cord, acting like a liquid shock absorber. It should contain no red blood cells, few white blood cells and only minute amounts of protein and glucose.

Because the CSF is in such direct contact with the brain, it is often tested when infectious diseases of the brain or nervous system, such as *meningitis* and *encephalitis* are suspected. A **VDRL Test** of the fluid can indicate the spread of *syphilis* to the nervous system. Blood in the fluid may help diagnose *stroke, hemmorhage* or *embolism*, and higher than usual fluid pressure may indicate infection or a *brain tumor*. Changes in the amount of protein and/or sugar help in diagnosing certain types of infections of the central nervous system. Though some of the above diagnostic functions are now being supplanted by **CAT Scanning**, a spinal tap remains essential in diagnosing infection.

A doctor performs the test, often in your own hospital room. You lie on your side in the fetal position, with your head bowed and clasping your knees. This position stretches the back, maximizing the space between the vertebrae. The fluid will be taken from the lower back (lumbar area). After it is cleansed, you will feel a sharp sting as a needle with local anesthetic numbs the area. This is followed by a longer needle. You should feel pressure now but no pain as the needle passes through skin, muscle and the dura membrane. Very rarely, the needle grazes a nerve giving you a sharp twinge in the leg or groin. If this should happen, the doctor will immediately reposition the needle. (The puncture site is well below the spinal cord itself, so the danger of permanent nerve damage is very slim.) The best thing you can do to avoid complications is to stay still, breathe steadily and try to relax as much as possible.

When the needle has penetrated the spinal column, a manometer is attached and a fluid pressure reading taken. The manometer is then replaced by a syringe and samples are collected. Pressure is measured one more time before the needle is withdrawn. Nothing more than a band-aid is needed to seal the puncture.

Samples of the fluid are immediately examined for color and clarity (cloudiness is an indication of infection) before being sent to the lab. If your physician suspects meningitis, the fluid will be stained, cultured and sensitivity tested to determine the causative agent and the drug best suited to combat it. Though complete results may take 36 hours, antibiotics are usually prescribed immediately.

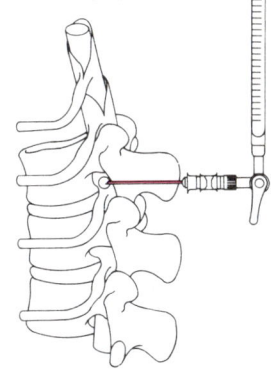

After the test you will be instructed to lie flat for 6 to 12 hours—the longer the better. This, and drinking fluids, will help reduce the severe headaches that can sometimes follow a spinal tap. Some people never get them, but if they do come, they usually don't last longer than a day or 2.

Meningitis *is an inflammation of the membranes that cover the brain and spinal cord. The infectious agent enters through the blood, respiratory system or as the result of a head wound. Rapid inflammation of the membranes ensues, and the space once filled with clear fluid fills with pus. Brain damage and death can follow. Fortunately,* bacterial meningitis *(70 percent of all cases) can be treated with antibiotics.*

Meningitis is most common in children, particularly those between 3 months and 2 years of age. The danger is compounded by an infant's inability to describe his or her symptoms. Things to look for include fever, headache and stiff neck. The child may become irritable, unusally withdrawn and sensitive to bright light. There also may be vomiting and swelling of the head. In both adults and children, the illness may show itself rapidly, within less than 24 hours. It is not unusual for a concerned doctor to order a spinal tap when an infant presents any of the above symptoms and an unexplained high fever.

109 STRESS TEST EXERCISE TOLERANCE TEST, TREADMILL TEST, STRESS EKG

The principle behind the test is simple. Coronary arteries that are blocked or narrowed may function adequately when you are at rest,

51

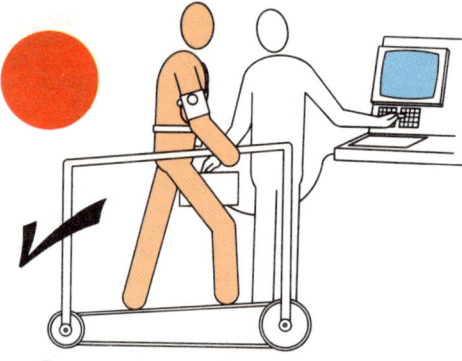

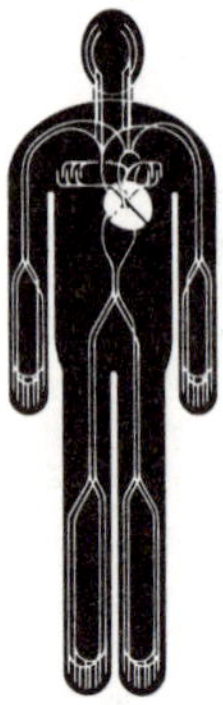

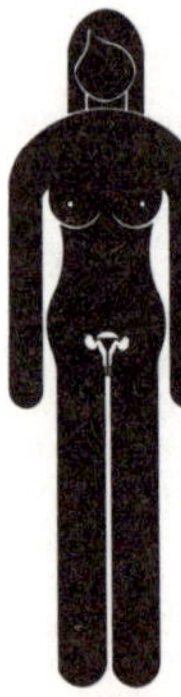

but during exertion they will be unable to meet the heart's increased need for oxygenated blood. This results in a characteristic change in the heart's electrical activity which can be read on an EKG tracing.

You should eat only a light breakfast that morning and refrain from coffee, alcohol and cigarettes for at least 4 hours before the test. You should report to the hospital or cardiologist's office in comfortable pants or shorts and should bring comfortable shoes, like sneakers.

A blood pressure cuff is wrapped around your arm and several electrodes are painlessly attached to your chest. EKG, heart rate and blood pressure readings are taken while you are at rest; then you begin slow and steady exercise on a moving treadmill or a stationary bicycle. While you are exercising, heart rate, blood pressure and EKG readings are continuously monitored and recorded. Because the object of the test is to put—under controlled conditions—strain on the heart sufficient to cause symptoms, the speed and or angle of the treadmill is increased every several minutes. You may also be asked to stop exercising momentarily and rest before resuming activity. If the physician notices any *distress, shortness of breath, irregular heart rhythms*, or if you report any chest pains (*angina*) the test is stopped. Otherwise, the test continues for a set period of time, usually about 20 minutes. Afterwards you rest for 5 to 15 minutes while more readings are recorded. You should then be free to leave.

A healthy person taking the test should experience little or no discomfort. However, a person with *coronary artery disease* or recovering from a *heart attack* may find it tiring and may experience the uncomfortable but transitory chest pains of *angina*. It is not a test of bravery. If you feel pain you must notify your physician immediately. There is a very small risk of *heart attack* or *arrhythmias* during stress testing, which is why the test is always performed under direct supervision of a cardiologist and in a place where the necessary emergency equipment is available.

110 SYPHILIS VDRL, FTA-ABS, WASSERMAN, DARK FIELD ILLUMINATION

Beethoven had it, so did Flaubert and Nietzsche. Some say even George Washington had it. Syphilis, the *French Pox*, was once the scourge of the Western world. Despite the fact that the disease can now be detected and cured easily, we mustn't forget that syphilis is very serious stuff. Symptoms may appear briefly and vanish, or they may imitate the symptoms of other ailments and go undiagnosed. Years after inception, an untreated case of syphilis may cause terrible damage to the heart, blood vessels, central nervous system and brain. It can damage any major organ of the body.

The symptoms of first stage syphilis are small, painless, open *sores* on the penis, vagina or rectum. They may be accompanied by local *swelling* in the lymph glands and *fever*. Within several weeks the disease enters its second stage. The sores usually clear up. The infected person may develop a *rash, sore throat, generalized swelling in the lymph glands, malaise* and *fever*—or he or she may have none of these symptoms. Your doctor may order a syphilis test if there is undiagnosed infection and any of the above symptoms. Syphilis is known as the *great masquerader,* the infection that can mimic or hide the symptoms of many other diseases.

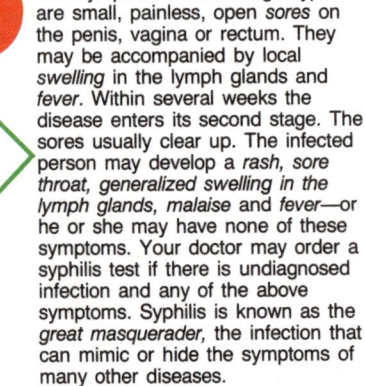

Syphilis can be cured with antibiotics and can be detected by at least a dozen different testing methods. The most common is a **VDRL (Venereal Disease Research Lab)** blood test. This test detects antibodies (the body's microscopic defense against invasion by foreign bacteria) that fight the tiny spiral-shaped microorganism that causes syphilis. Though a VDRL is probably the test most commonly prescribed, it is basically a screening test. A patient with *hepatitis, mononucleosis* or *pneumonia* may have false positive results. Confirmation of syphilis is done with another more specific and slightly more expensive test called **FTA-ABS**. In some cases the 2 tests are done simultaneously. Syphilis can also be detected by **Dark Field Illumination**—culturing a sore and examining the sample under a microscope for direct presence of the spirochete (a delicate spiral bacterium).

Almost all states require that pregnant women and couples about to marry have a blood test for syphilis. Most patients with gonorrhea are also routinely tested for syphilis. Patients with syphilis are often retested after treatment to make sure the infection is gone. Though not all doctors comply in many states they are required to report all syphilis cases to a public health office. You may then be visited by a public health official who will request the names of your sexual contacts so they can be notified and tested. It is policy to preserve your anonymity.

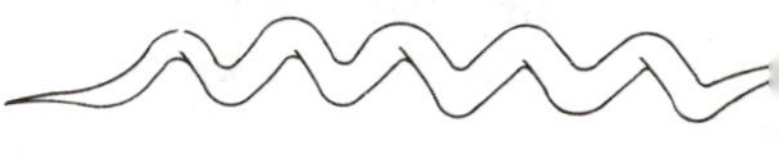

111 TEMPERATURE

The body's internal temperature is carefully regulated by the brain which keeps it basically constant at 98.6 degrees F (37 degrees C). Any large change in temperature is therefore very significant. High temperature or fever is often the first outward sign of infection. It is your body's automatic response to invasion by bacteria or viruses. Infection fighting white blood cells work better at high temperatures and in some cases the heat alone may be enough to kill the invading organism. However, if fever rises above 102 degrees F, the therapeutic effects are outweighed by the heat damage to various organs and the fever must be treated.

Several kinds of thermometers are available, the glass and mercury kind, paper strips that record temperature by color change and electric thermometers with a digital readout. This last is fast becoming the most popular type in hospitals. A plastic sleeve can easily be put over the tip to ensure sterility and an accurate reading takes only 15 seconds. In almost all cases, temperature is taken orally. However, rectal readings are taken in small children, unconscious patients or patients whose severe shortness of breath prevents them from keeping the thermometer in their mouth.

*Temperature is one of the 4 **vital signs** (along with respiratory rate, blood pressure and pulse) that must be checked regularly in very ill patients or those recovering from surgery. If the surgery was a long one and risk of infection greater, your temperature will be checked more frequently.*

There is no medical evidence to indicate that Feed a cold; starve a fever *is a correct approach.*

112 THERMOGRAPHY

Two thousand years ago Hippocrates spread an even coating of clay over his patients and observed that some parts of the body dried faster than others. He reasoned, correctly, that the quick drying parts corresponded to internal disease or injury. It was primitive but essentially the same principle used in modern thermography. Certain diseased parts of the body, particularly *malignant tumors*, tend to have greater blood flow or metabolic activity and hence give off more heat than other parts. Recently thermography has been used in diagnosis of *tumors, whiplash, blood clots, gangrene* and *nonspecific pain* in the head, neck and back. Thermography has also been used to determine whether *male impotence* is due to psychological or physical causes.

The technique is simple, painless and free from radiation exposure. You undress or expose the part of the body in question and wait for a few moments while the body adjusts to room temperature. Then the thermographic system begins scanning, a process that takes about a minute. The unit used in most hospitals resembles a TV camera. At its heart are semiconductor chips sensitive to infrared energy. They send signals to a computer which converts the information into colorful graphic or video images that look somewhat like topographic maps with each heat contour in a different color. Abnormalities show up as hot spots. To ensure accuracy, several sets of pictures are usually taken at 20-minute intervals. The results are available the same day.

In the early 70s, thermography was heralded as a possible breakthrough tool for early diagnosis of breast cancer. While some physicians recommend it because it is risk-free, mainstream medical thought now maintains that thermography is not accurate enough to be a primary diagnostic or screening test for breast cancer. The American college of Radiology states as its policy that **Ultrasound, Thermography** and transillumination must be regarded as experimental techniques in breast cancer detection and that self-examination and x-ray **Mammography** are the only approved screening methods.

113 THROAT CULTURE

A sore throat (the technical term is *pharyngitis*) can be caused by any number of bacteria or viruses. When the doctor uses a tongue depressor and looks into your mouth, he or she can see redness and pus on the tonsils or back of the throat, but can't tell what is causing the infection. His or her primary concern is that you don't have *strep throat*, an infection caused by the *streptoccocus* bacterium. Only 5 percent of adults with sore throats have strep, but it is very common in children. Although strep throat responds when treated with antibiotics, untreated strep can, in rare instances, lead to *nephritis*, an inflammation of the kidneys, or *rheumatic fever*, an infection that may affect the joints and heart tissue, in some cases leaving lasting damage.

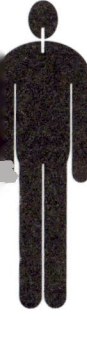

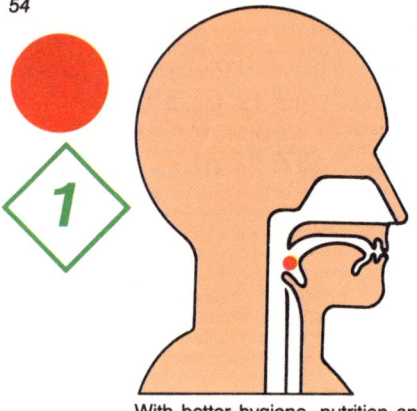

With better hygiene, nutrition and the advent of antibiotics, rheumatic fever has become very rare. Doctors' policies on throat cultures vary: some doctors are eager to take a throat culture whenever there is a sore throat; others only order one when other strep symptoms, such as *fever, pus* and *swollen lymph glands*, are also present.

Either the doctor or nurse may take the culture. You open your mouth wide and a sterile swab (basically an extra long cotton swab) is rubbed over the back of the throat to get a good sample of whatever is there. It is quick and painless, though many patients gag momentarily. The sample is sent to a lab to be cultured at a constant 98.6 degrees F. This provides optimal conditions for any bacteria present to grow. The sample is microscopically examined for streptoccocus bacteria. If strep is found there is no need for further testing. Strep infections respond to penicillin and other antibiotics.

114 THYROID FUNCTION TESTS

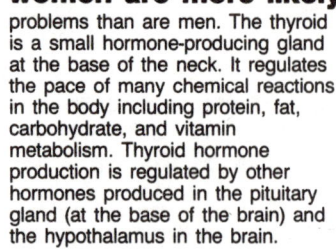

Thyroid disorders are fairly common. Up to 5 percent of the population is affected, and women are more likely to develop thyroid problems than are men. The thyroid is a small hormone-producing gland at the base of the neck. It regulates the pace of many chemical reactions in the body including protein, fat, carbohydrate, and vitamin metabolism. Thyroid hormone production is regulated by other hormones produced in the pituitary gland (at the base of the brain) and the hypothalamus in the brain.

Disorders of the thyroid may present several, often overlapping, symptoms and can have several underlying causes. The most common dysfunctions may cause metabolic changes like *lethargy* and *weight gain* or *nervousness* and *weight loss* if hormone levels are too high or too low. These changes may or may not be accompanied by physical changes in the gland itself such as swelling or the development of nodules. Nodules are isolated areas of enlargement that are usually benign, but testing is required to make sure. Fortunately cancer of the thyroid is slow growing and when treated early has a cure rate of more than 90 percent.

Though there are standard textbook symptoms of thyroid dysfunction, symptoms can be mild and easily attributed to other causes. Therefore, a series of tests is usually required to establish that there is an abnormality as well as its cause. Hypothyroidism, for example, could be caused by *primary thyroid disease*, where the body's own immune system attacks the gland, *infection, iodine deficiency* or an underlying problem in the brain that affects the pituitary gland.

The thyroid function tests comprise the first step of diagnosis. They are a series of tests performed on a single blood sample. The patient experience is simple, a plain needle prick, but the lab procedures required to isolate the various hormones are quite complex and usually cost a bit more than most lab tests. There are at least 5 possible tests that may be done on the blood sample, though your doctor will probably not have to order all of them. After a hormone level abnormality has been established, further testing may be needed, for instance to determine if the abnormality is caused by a benign or cancerous growth. These tests may include **Ultrasound, Radioactive iodine uptake (104)** and a **Thyroid scan (104).** Most thyroid conditions can be controlled with synthetic thyroid hormone or antithyroid medication, however, those on medication may require regular blood testing to assure correct dosage.

115 TONOMETRY

Tonometry is the basic screening test for *glaucoma*, **a condition which causes irreversible eye damage and is the leading cause of** blindness in people over 40. Though there may be warning signs—*eye pain, blurry vision, headaches*—glaucoma typically presents no symptoms until the damage has already begun. For that reason, regular testing by your personal physician or eye doctor is strongly recommended, every 2 or 3 years for adults over 40, as often as once a year if there is a family history of glaucoma.

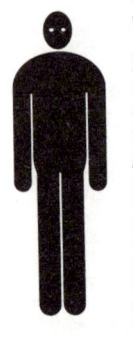

Glaucoma is caused by a gradual build-up of fluid pressure inside the eye. Glaucoma can be detected early by measuring the increase in fluid pressure inside the eye (*intraocular pressure*) that causes it. Measuring this intraocular pressure is called tonometry. There are several different methods, all are safe and painless.

The most common test uses a *Schiotz tonometer*, a delicate mechanical device that measures the eye's resistance to slight pressure applied to the surface of the eyeball.

1

The test can be performed in the hospital or a doctor's office. The lights are usually lowered and you are instructed to loosen ties or tight collars. You lie down or recline with your head back. Several drops of anesthetic are put in the eyes. They should start working within 30 seconds. You stare straight up at the ceiling while the tonometer is moved over the eye. The footplate, which provides a stable base, is brought to rest on the cornea. A plunger inside the footplate rests on the exact center of the eye. The eye's resistance to this slight pressure is measured on a gauge connected to the other end of the plunger.

First 1 eye is tested, then the other. The test isn't painful, but many patients find it difficult to remain still. There is a very small chance that the cornea will be scratched. This is very rare and the cornea usually heals without incident.

Non-contact tonometry is another method used to measure intraocular pressure. You sit on one side of the non-contact tonometer with your head and chin positioned by supports. A doctor or technician sits on the other side. The machine shines a focused beam of light at the eye. Then, at the operator's command, a small puff of air is directed toward the cornea of the eye. The force of the air is gradually increased until the surface of the cornea flattens and redirects the beam of light into a light detector. The pressure reading is taken by analyzing how much air pressure is required to redirect the beam of light. First 1 eye is tested, then the other. The whole procedure takes about 10 minutes and is painless.

When tonometry is done as part of a complete exam in an ophthalmologist's office, a slit lamp may be used. You place your chin on a chin rest while the doctor focuses a light on the eye and looks at it through an eyepiece. He or she controls a small prism or probe which touches the surface of the eye for an instant and notes the moment when sufficient pressure to flatten the cornea has been applied. The results of all types of tonometry are available immediately.

The **aqueous humor** *is clear fluid that circulates between the cornea and the iris, bathing the lens. In a healthy eye this fluid is produced and drained off at a constant rate. In glaucoma the fluid drains too slowly or not at all. Pressure builds up in the front of the eye. This pressure is exerted through the lens to the* **vitreous humor***, the jelly-like fluid that fills the rear part of the eyeball. Excessive pressure in the rear of the eye causes the collapse of the tiny blood vessels that nourish the retina and the optic nerve. Deprived of nourishment, they gradually die and vision is lost. Frequently one eye is affected and then the other. Fortunately, when glaucoma is detected early, it can be successfully treated with medication.*

Non-Contact Tonometry

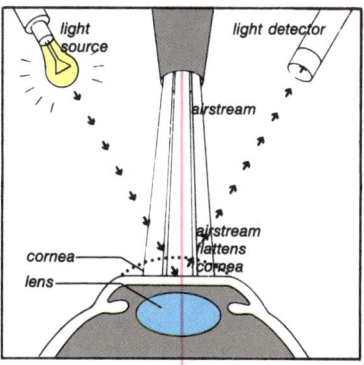

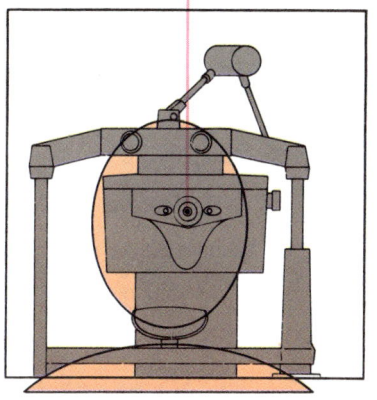

116 TUBERCULOSIS SKIN TEST *PPD, TINE TEST, TB TEST*

A very common screening test, but not a particularly accurate one. The test does not distinguish between someone who has an active

case of tuberculosis and someone who was exposed a long while ago and who now harbors a dormant infection. Children are the most frequently tested, at 1, 3 and 5 years of age.

A very small amount of dead tuberculosis bacteria is injected into the skin causing a small raised whitish bump. It is checked over the next 48-72 hours for signs of *swelling*, *redness* and *itching*, which indicate whether you have been previously exposed to tuberculosis. The only important finding is swelling. (If you have been immunized with BCG, *bacillus Calmette-Guérin*, a cow tuberculosis vaccine, you will have a false positive reaction.) You cannot contract tuberculosis from the test.

The test is usually done with either a small needle or a *tine,* a little white button with 4 tiny protruding needles. It's quickly pressed into the skin of the arm or shoulder. There is a brief sting, but it hurts much less than a regular injection.

If the doctor suspects active tuberculosis, a chest x-ray and a sample of sputum will be taken and cultured. Sputum is not saliva. It is the mucosal secretions found deep in the airways and lungs. A patient can bring it up by deep coughing.

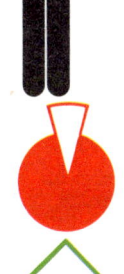

117 UPPER GI SMALL BOWEL SERIES

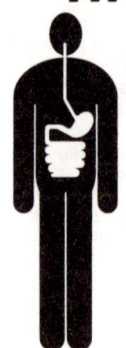

An upper GI is a fairly common, and not too trying, x-ray study used to evaluate the first part of the digestive tract which includes the

esophagus, stomach, duodenum and the small intestine. Because these soft tissues of the body do not show up well on conventional x-rays, you must first drink a *barium cocktail* or *milkshake*, a large cupful of a thick, white, chalky liquid. The barium coats the inside of the digestive tract and allows its contours and any irregularities to be seen on x-rays. The test may be used to diagnose *ulcers, tumors* (either inside the digestive tract or pressing on it from outside), *inflammation, hiatal hernia* and *swallowing disorders of the esophagus*. It may also be used to assess how well ulcers are healing. The test may be ordered if you are experiencing *abdominal pain,* what feels like *severe indigestion, unexplained vomiting,* or if an **Occult blood test** of your stool has indicated that you are *bleeding internally*.

The test is often done on an outpatient basis. Though it can be tedious, it is minimally discomforting. You fast—no liquids or solid food—for 8 hours before the test and then report to a hospital radiology department where you are given the barium to drink. Though flavoring is often added, it's hardly what you would call delicious. When the test begins you are either lying on an x-ray table or leaning against an upright table that will be tilted back during the course of the exam. The progress of the barium is watched on a **fluoroscope**, a machine that takes moving x-ray pictures and shows them on a TV screen; still x-rays are taken intermittently. In some cases a doctor presses on your abdomen to get better barium distribution. This may be mildly uncomfortable. The duration of the test depends on how much of you they want to see. If ulcers are suspected in the stomach, the test may only last for half an hour. If, however, the entire small intestine must be visualized, you may have to stay in the radiology department for up to 4 hours.

You should be able to go home and resume a normal diet immediately after the study. You will probably be constipated for a couple of days afterwards. You will probably be told to increase your fluid intake and you may be given a laxative to hasten the expulsion of the barium. Stool is typically light-colored or even white for 24 to 72 hours.

118 URINALYSIS

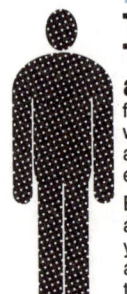

The kidneys' principal role is waste removal. They receive about 25 percent of cardiac output a minute, that is approximately 200 quarts of

filtered blood a day. The collected wastes and excess salts and water are excreted in urine (about a quart every 24 hours).

Because the urine is so readily available and an analysis of it can yield a great deal of information about overall health, and the health of the kidneys in particular, **Urinalysis** is part of every complete physical.

While there are many tests that may be done on urine (**Electrolytes, Bilirubin,** hormones, mineral and drug levels), this entry only discusses the tests that are commonly conducted in a routine urinalysis. Many of the following tests can be done in a doctor's office in minutes with the aid of *dipsticks*. These are small strips of paper or plastic that have been coated in bands with reactive chemicals that change color in the presence of certain other chemicals in the urine. The person performing the test puts the dipstick in the urine specimen and then compares the color of the various bands with a standardized chart. Home testing kits with dipsticks and charts are now available in many pharmacies.

In most cases a random sample of urine in a dry sterile container is all that's needed. If it won't be analyzed within an hour, it should be refrigerated. If you're in the hospital, samples are requested in the morning when urine concentration is high and bacteria most active. Routine urinalysis includes:

Visual examination. Urine is usually clear and ranges in color from straw to amber. Any blood or cloudiness is significant. Certain drugs and diseases can change the color to bright orange, black and even blue. Pink is usually an indication of blood in the urine. Cloudy urine is often a sign of infection and brownish urine may indicate excessive bilirubin caused by liver disease.

Specific gravity. This is a measure of the proportion of dissolved material to total volume. It indicates the ability of the kidney to concentrate and dilute fluid.

pH. pH refers to how acid or alkaline your urine is. Urine may be acidic in cases of *diabetes* or *dehydration*. Highly alkaline (low in acid) urine is present where there is a *urinary tract infection, aspirin overdose,* certain types of *kidney disease* and a diet high in citrus.

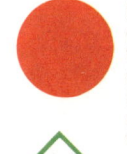

Glucose (sugar). There should be no glucose in the urine. When there is, it often means that the sugar level in blood entering the kidney is so high it exceeds the kidney's ability to pass it back into the blood. The spillover ends up in the urine. The condition is associated with *diabetes* but is also common in *pancreatitis* and *hypothyroidism*. Glucose testing is a common screening test used to detect diabetes. It may also be done frequently on a newly diagnosed patient when monitoring the effectiveness of treatment. Glucose levels may be tested at home with a dipstick.

Ketones are a by-product of fat metabolism. If the body is starved or can't make use of blood sugar in a normal way, in *diabetes* for instance, it is forced to metabolize stored fat. Ketones spill over from the blood into the urine. This may happen in *uncontrolled diabetes, malnutrition, starvation, or excessive dieting*. Ketones may also be present in cases of *fever* or *aspirin overdose*.

Hemoglobin. Urine is tested for hemoglobin, a product of broken down blood, as well as for whole blood cells. Hemoglobin in urine may indicate *kidney disease* or a problem in the lining of the urinary system. A kidney stone for instance, could scrape the lining and put hemoglobin in the urine. It is not uncommon to have some blood in the urine after exertion like jogging or football.

Nitrite. Many of the bacteria that cause urinary infections convert nitrate to nitrite as they multiply. A positive nitrite test is a good indication of infection.

Protein. A functioning kidney does not allow protein molecules to pass through, so there should be no protein in the urine. Many doctors consider this to be one of the best early warning signs of kidney disease. However, people with a fever or who have just recently engaged in very strenuous physical activity may have trace amounts of protein in the blood. It is a common finding, for instance in boxers and marathon runners.

Microscopic analysis. A small amount of urine is examined under a microscope, usually after the sample has been spun at high speed to separate the liquid from any solid matter. The sediment is examined for red blood cells, white blood cells, bacteria and crystals. Red blood cells typically indicate some kind of *kidney disease* or *trauma*. White blood cells are present when there is a *urinary infection*. Crystals form in the urine as it cools. Their presence often indicates that *kidney stones* already exist or are forming.

Urine culture. If bacteria are present under the microscope or you report symptoms such as *frequent urination* and *pain* or *burning* upon urination, your doctor may suspect a urinary tract infection and order a urine culture. In this case, a **clean catch** or **midstream specimen** is needed, i.e., a specimen that is uncontaminated by bacteria from the genitals or the first part of the urethra. You are given swabs and an antiseptic and instructed on how to clean the genitals. You begin urination in the toilet and then stop and position a sterile container so that the rest of the sample may be collected. The sample is then sent to a lab where special preparations help foster the growth of any bacteria that are present so that they can be identified and treated.

119 VENOGRAPHY *VENOGRAM*

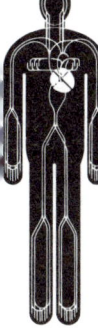

Venography is used to evaluate the veins of the leg and detect any blockages or blood clots that might later dislodge and lead to a more dangerous blockage elsewhere in the body. Contrast material is injected in a vein in the leg and several x-rays are taken. The test may be ordered when symptoms such as *pain* or *swelling* indicate *thrombophlebitis* or when *chest pain* and *shortness of breath* suggest that a *clot fragment* has already broken off and traveled to the lungs. **Doppler ultrasound** and **Plethysmography** are other noninvasive tests that may help get the same information, but they tend to be less accurate.

No advance preparation is needed. You change into a gown in a hospital radiology department and lie on an x-ray table, usually one that can be tilted 180 degrees into an upright position. An area low on the leg near the ankle is cleansed and a needle is inserted in a vein. In some instances a small incision must be made to locate a vein. When the iodine-based dye is injected, you may feel a brief burning sensation all over your body and perhaps some nausea, but this usually passes within a minute. The needle insertion and dye injection may be somewhat painful, particularly if the vein is badly inflamed. If your physician anticipates this to be the case, you may be given a sedative before the test.

The exam continues in 1 of 2 ways. A tourniquet is wrapped around the leg to control the flow of dye; or, while you stand on one leg, the table is tilted until you are almost upright. Gravity then assures that the dye is evenly distributed. The upward movement of the dye is traced on a *flouroscope*, a machine that takes moving x-ray pictures, and several still x-rays are taken for permanent record. After the x-rays are taken, a saltwater solution may be injected through the needle to help clear the veins of dye. The site of insertion is then closed with a few stitches if an incision was used, or bandaged if no incision was necessary. You are watched closely for an hour or so to make sure there is no bleeding at the insertion site, no allergic reaction to the dye and that the force of the dye injection or pressure from the tourniquet has not caused a clot to break loose, a possible but rare complication. The test lasts from 30 minutes to an hour. If you are not already hospitalized, you should be able to return home the same day. As with all tests that require injection of iodine-based contrast dye, an allergic reaction is possible. You must inform your doctor of any allergies, particularly to iodine or seafood which is high in iodine.

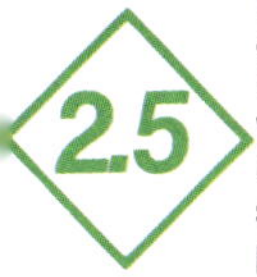

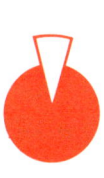

120 VISUAL ACUITY EYE TEST, SNELLEN CHART

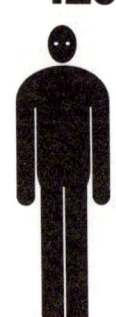

Even if nothing seems wrong with your eyes, it is recommended that your vision be checked regularly. Almost every private physician has an eye chart hanging on the office wall and a quick glance at it is routinely included in a complete physical. Children should be tested at age 5 before they enter school and again at age 12 which is when farsightedness tends to make itself evident. Adults over 40 should be tested regularly to detect progressive eye problems associated with aging.

The visual acuity (sharpness) test, the most common eye exam, measures how near and far you can see. No special preparation is needed and it can be performed in any well-lit area where you can stand 20 feet away from the chart. The Snellen chart, still in use today, was invented by a Dutch optometrist in 1862. It has several rows of letters and numbers in gradually decreasing size. For children and others who can't read, new charts are available that show pictures of animals or common household objects.

If you wear glasses, you'll be asked to bring them with you. To begin the examination, you will face the chart at a distance of 20 feet. Without your glasses, and with 1 eye covered, you will be asked to identify the letters, numbers or symbols pointed to by the examiner. You will also be asked to read the smallest line of print that you can. This same procedure will be repeated while you cover your other eye. Finally, the test will be repeated while you wear your glasses in order to determine how well they correct your vision.

Having determined the smallest line of print you can read (half the letters or more), the examiner will record your visual acuity as a fraction (e.g., 20/40). The top number indicates the distance at which you read the letters (usually 20 feet), and the bottom number, the distance at which a normal eye can read that same line of letters. The results may be different for each eye.

Vision of 20/200 means that a person can read at 20 feet only the very large letters, which a person with normal vision can read at 200 feet. The larger the bottom number in the fraction, the worse the vision. Sometimes the fraction is followed by the word *corrected,* meaning that a person can read a particular line while wearing glasses. While normal vision is designated as 20/20, vision up to 20/40 without the aid of glasses is still considered satisfactory.

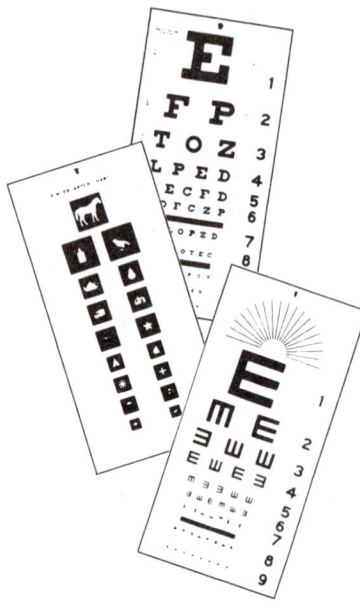

This test is fine for detecting nearsightedness *(myopia)*, in which one can easily read or see nearby objects but not far ones, and farsightedness *(hyperopia)* in which the reverse is true. It is not, however, precise enough to determine a prescription for glasses. For that, further testing is required, usually at the office of an *ophthalmologist* or *optometrist.*

Ophthalmologists are physicians who specialize in treating eye disorders and performing eye surgery. They prescribe glasses, contact lenses and drugs. Optometrists are not physicians; they are trained to test vision and prescribe glasses or contacts. Opticians fit glasses and lenses according to the prescriptions of ophthalmologists and optometrists.

A person with normal vision can distinguish a letter 3/8 inch high from 20 feet away. Such vision is recorded as 20/20.

The big E on the Snellen chart is 3 1/2 inches high. The legal definition of blindness is 20/200 or worse, with the use of corrective lenses.

When you blink, about 25 times a minute, the eyelids wash the surface of the eye with lubricating tears.

TERMS

Accuracy. No test is 100 percent accurate. Drugs may alter the result, a sample may be left out too long and deteriorate, machines can be miscalibrated, but above and beyond all that, each test has a statistical margin of error. Tests are rated on *sensitivity* and *specificity.* Sensitivity refers to a test's ability to detect an abnormality if it is present, and specificity refers to its ability to detect only that abnormality and not be fooled into giving a false positive result because of other factors. Certain home use kits, which test the stool for blood, for instance, are very sensitive, but not specific. If you eat red meat, certain vegetables or take iron supplements, you might come back with a positive result. Your doctor should be familiar with the accuracy of the tests prescribed and be prepared to discuss the matter with you.

Angiography. Any study of the arteries that requires an injection of dye to make them show up well on x-ray film. Blood vessels in the heart, head, lung and kidney are among those that can be studied this way. Angiographic tests are invasive.

Biopsy. This refers to removal of a tiny bit of tissue for microscopic examination, usually to determine if the tissue is cancerous. The sample can be taken from almost anywhere and by a number of different methods. Tissue may be removed during surgery or during tests like **Bronchoscopy** and **Gastroscopy**. A biopsy is considered invasive.

Contrast material. In order to make certain organs visible on x-rays, a contrast material or radiopaque dye must be used. In a **Barium enema,** for instance, a thick liquid is passed through the rectum into the large intestine which then shows up as a clear outline on x-ray film. In other studies, a dye that shows up strongly on x-rays is injected into the blood stream or sometimes infused through a catheter (small hollow tube) that has been inserted into a blood vessel. This contrast material is usually iodine-based and can provoke a strong allergic reaction called *anaphylaxis* in patients who are allergic to iodine. Before any contrast study, make sure your doctor knows about any allergies you might have, particularly to iodine or to seafood which is high in iodine. In many cases premedication can prevent any adverse reaction. Contrast x-rays are more uncomfortable than regular x-rays (the dye makes some people feel flushed and nauseous) and usually require a consent form.

Culture. The purpose of a culture is to discover if illness is caused by a microorganism, and if so, which one. Blood, urine, spinal fluid, pus from the back of the throat and discharge from the urethra can all be cultured. How the sample is taken varies from test to test, but the lab procedure is the same. The sample is put in a container with nutrients and kept at 98.6 degrees Fahrenheit. Within 24 to 48 hours, any bacteria present will have multiplied and become identifiable. The bacteria may then be exposed to several antibiotics to determine which drug is most effective in killing it. This is called *sensitivity testing.*

Endoscopy. Endoscopic or scoping procedures use long, often flexible, tubes to see inside the body. Fiberoptic bundles inside the scope carry light to the area under investigation as well as an image back to the physician's eyepiece. Minute cable-controlled tools can be passed through the tube and used to stop bleeding, remove growths and retrieve samples for biopsy. The inside of the lungs, stomach, bladder and colon are just some of the areas that can be examined by endoscopy. Most scoping procedures are done while the patient is awake. Endoscopic procedures are invasive and require a consent form.

Fluoroscopy. This is a technique that makes moving x-ray pictures that are shown on a TV monitor and may be recorded for later reference. Fluoroscopy is frequently used when guiding catheters inside the body and when watching the progress of injected contrast materials.

Normal is a relative word in medical testing. The normal ranges for any one test vary from lab to lab. They certainly vary from person to person, according to age, sex and weight. Also, some doctors may have a personal view of what are acceptable normal values. In any event, what you must discuss with your doctor is his or her interpretation, not the numbers.

Nuclear medicine. Nuclear studies, also called nuclear scans or radionuclide imaging, use something called radioisotopes to help visualize internal organs, evaluate their function and size and distinguish between normal and abnormal tissue. Radioisotopes are chemicals exposed to very low levels of radiation and then injected into the body. Each radioisotope is chosen for its tendency to concentrate in a specific organ such as bone or liver. You receive the isotope by mouth or injection and after a suitable time has elapsed, the organ in question is scanned by a special camera that may be called a *gamma camera,* a *rectilinear scanner* or a *scintillation camera.* Working like a Geiger counter, it detects the pattern of radiation distribution and translates that informaton into an image. The radiation used in nuclear tests is low dosage; exposure compares favorably with conventional x-rays. These scans are not available everywhere, but they are becoming increasingly popular for diagnosing ailments of the thyroid, bone and liver. They are not usually recommended for pregnant or nursing mothers.

Screening. These tests are usually simple and inexpensive. They are used for early detection of common ailments in people who are healthy and report no symptoms. **Urinalysis, Pap smears** and **Blood glucose** are all screening tests. Screening tests tend to be less accurate (more likely to produce a false positive) than other tests. Though they may alert your doctor to a problem, a diagnosis should be based on more precise tests.

X-rays. A type of electromagnetic radiation (like light) whose wave length is short enough to pass through certain objects. The denser the object, the less x-rays pass through it. Bones, which are very dense, show up as a strong white shadow on x-ray film. X-rays pass right through the gas-filled lungs which show up as black. While newer equipment has reduced the risks of radiation to very acceptable limits, there are things you can do to further lessen the risk. Try to get your x-rays taken on the newest equipment. Make sure you are given a lead shield to protect your reproductive organs. Remain still during the x-ray so the image is good and more x-rays aren't needed. Try not to repeat x-ray tests when previous x-rays will provide the needed information. X-rays are not usually performed on pregnant women unless they are absolutely necessary.

From Blepharoplasty to Bunion removal, Facelifts to Fractures, some aspects of surgery are common to most procedures.

Standard Activities and Procedures.

Certain measures are fairly standard in the care of all surgical patients. These procedures are routinely performed, but in the case of an emergency patient whose condition requires immediate surgical intervention, there may not be enough time to wait for all of the test results before operating. However, these studies will be carried out and the results documented.

At admission, your temperature, pulse and respiration rates are recorded. Thereafter, your pulse and respirations are recorded at least once on every nursing shift as part of routine nursing care.

Your blood pressure is recorded shortly after admission, and again as part of the preoperative preparation. If you have a history or evidence of elevated blood pressure, it is usually recorded at least once on each nursing shift.

Tests and studies before surgery.

Most hospitals have established sets of preoperative diagnostic tests and studies that are performed for *all patients* scheduled for surgery. These studies must be specifically ordered by the physician, even though they are fairly standard. They are likely to include: **Complete blood count (CBC)**, **SMA 12, 16 or 26** (a set of 12, 16 or 26 different blood studies that can be performed on one blood sample), **Urinalysis**, **Chest x-ray** and **Electrocardiogram (ECG or EKG)** in patients over 39 years old. In a few local governmental jurisdictions, a **Syphilis** test may be required by law. Depending on the type of operation planned, certain other studies may be ordered.

If you have a history of excessive bleeding, or show a tendency to bleed profusely from minor injuries, coagulation or **Blood clotting tests (PT, PTT)** may be performed before surgery. If the results of this test show that your blood fails to clot normally, your surgery will be postponed until the clotting mechanism has been corrected, usually through transfusion with a blood component called *platelets*.

If extensive surgery associated with significant blood loss is planned, your blood will be *typed* and *cross matched* in case transfusion becomes necessary. Blood loss during surgery is closely monitored. If surgical blood loss exceeds an acceptable level, usually specified as around 300 cubic centimeters in an adult with a normal preoperative hemoglobin level, you will be transfused with the previously cross matched blood.

In nonemergency, planned surgery, you will probably have these studies performed before you are admitted to the hospital. Most insurance and employee benefit plans, as well as Medicare, will refuse to pay for a preoperative hospital stay if the preoperative testing. (An exception is made where the planned operation requires special preparations under direct medical supervision in a hospital.)

Nursing care plan.

The hospital's nursing service has developed a number of standard nursing care plans to be used as guides in the care of specific types of patients. Thus, it usually has 1 care plan for patients undergoing eye surgery, another for normal labor and delivery, another for patients who are having breast surgery. A nurse will interview you and evaluate your condition with reference to any special care that you may need after surgery. At this time, the nurse *customizes* the appropriate care plan. If you are not sent to your room until after surgery, the same evaluation takes place after the operation. During the evaluation interview, the nurse also instructs you in relevant procedures. You will be shown how to use the call system and told whether or not you may get out of bed. You will be asked about your diet and given any instructions from your physician.

Anesthesiologist's evaluation.

There are 2 types of professionals who administer the anesthetic: an anesthesiologist or an anesthetist. An anesthesiologist is a physician while an anesthetist is usually a registered nurse with special training in the administration of anesthesia. (If an anesthetist is going to administer the anesthetic, find out if an anesthesiologist MD will be on call nearby in the hospital.)

The day or night before your surgery, an anesthesiologist (MD) will visit you. You cannot choose an anesthesiologist in the same way as you can choose your physician. But, before your surgery, you should ask your physician about anesthesia and the quality of the anesthesiologists at his or her hospital or ambulatory care facility. Sometimes a surgeon will request a particular anesthesiologist to be assigned to your case; similarly, a surgeon may request not to work with a certain anesthesiologist. However, it is the anesthesiologist, not the surgeon, who will make the decision as to which type of anesthesia to use for your operation, based on the nature of the surgery and the overall condition of your health.

Anesthesia literally means *loss of sensation*. Four types of anesthesia are used depending on the type of operation and your particular condition.

1. **General anesthetic** makes you completely unconscious during the operation and can be administered by inhaling gas or by an intravenous injection (IV), usually through the vein on the back of your hand. If it is to be inhaled, it may be through a mask or through a tube inserted through your mouth into your windpipe. The tube is inserted only after you are asleep from a local IV injection so you will not feel it going down your throat. General anesthesia is most often used for major surgery. Surgery will not begin until you are completely asleep. Sometimes muscle relaxants are also given to reduce the amount of general anesthetic needed.

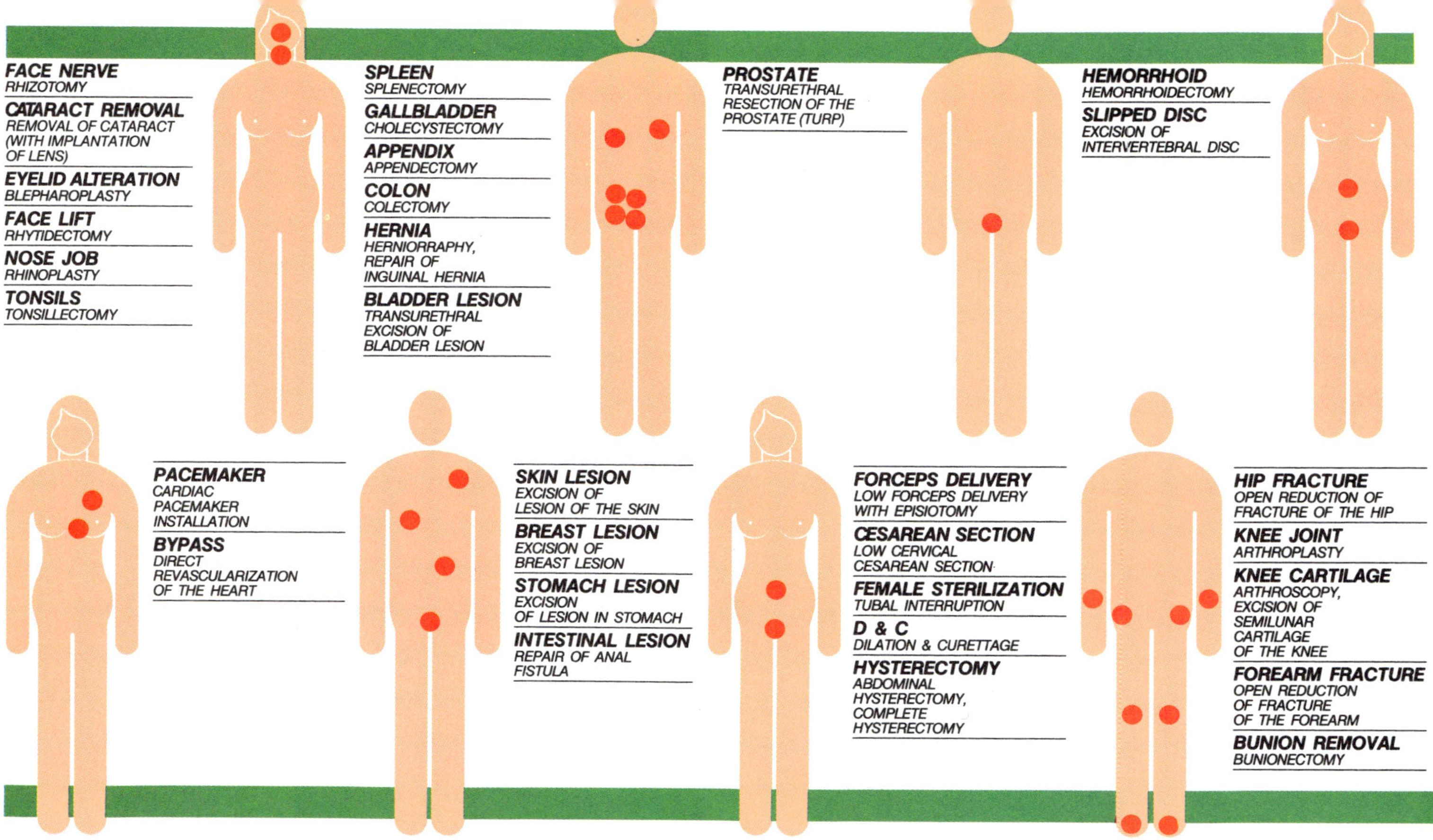

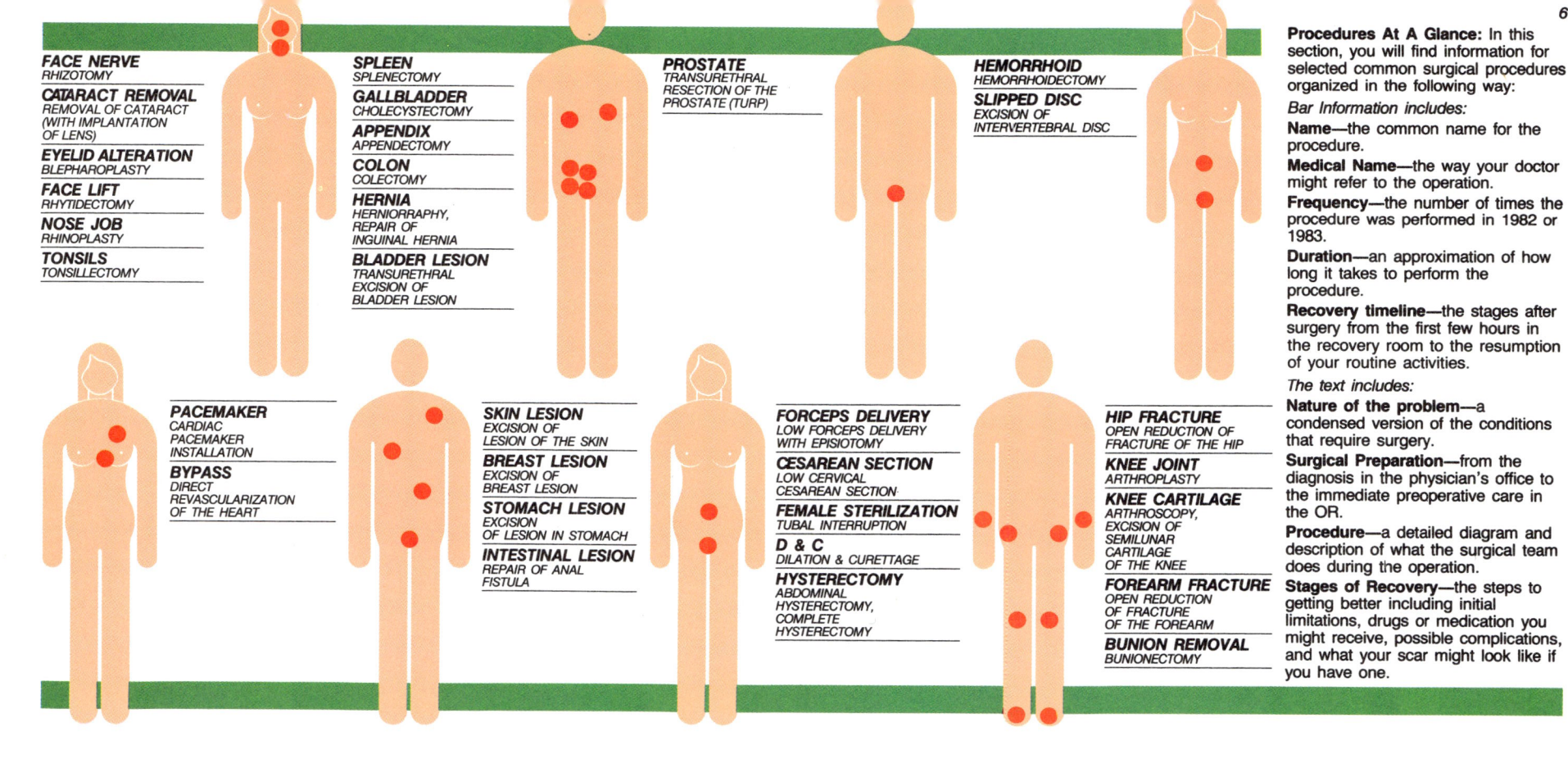

Procedures At A Glance: In this section, you will find information for selected common surgical procedures organized in the following way:

Bar Information includes:

Name—the common name for the procedure.

Medical Name—the way your doctor might refer to the operation.

Frequency—the number of times the procedure was performed in 1982 or 1983.

Duration—an approximation of how long it takes to perform the procedure.

Recovery timeline—the stages after surgery from the first few hours in the recovery room to the resumption of your routine activities.

The text includes:

Nature of the problem—a condensed version of the conditions that require surgery.

Surgical Preparation—from the diagnosis in the physician's office to the immediate preoperative care in the OR.

Procedure—a detailed diagram and description of what the surgical team does during the operation.

Stages of Recovery—the steps to getting better including initial limitations, drugs or medication you might receive, possible complications, and what your scar might look like if you have one.

FACE NERVE
RHIZOTOMY

CATARACT REMOVAL
REMOVAL OF CATARACT (WITH IMPLANTATION OF LENS)

EYELID ALTERATION
BLEPHAROPLASTY

FACE LIFT
RHYTIDECTOMY

NOSE JOB
RHINOPLASTY

TONSILS
TONSILLECTOMY

SPLEEN
SPLENECTOMY

GALLBLADDER
CHOLECYSTECTOMY

APPENDIX
APPENDECTOMY

COLON
COLECTOMY

HERNIA
HERNIORRAPHY, REPAIR OF INGUINAL HERNIA

BLADDER LESION
TRANSURETHRAL EXCISION OF BLADDER LESION

PROSTATE
TRANSURETHRAL RESECTION OF THE PROSTATE (TURP)

HEMORRHOID
HEMORRHOIDECTOMY

SLIPPED DISC
EXCISION OF INTERVERTEBRAL DISC

PACEMAKER
CARDIAC PACEMAKER INSTALLATION

BYPASS
DIRECT REVASCULARIZATION OF THE HEART

SKIN LESION
EXCISION OF LESION OF THE SKIN

BREAST LESION
EXCISION OF BREAST LESION

STOMACH LESION
EXCISION OF LESION IN STOMACH

INTESTINAL LESION
REPAIR OF ANAL FISTULA

FORCEPS DELIVERY
LOW FORCEPS DELIVERY WITH EPISIOTOMY

CESAREAN SECTION
LOW CERVICAL CESAREAN SECTION

FEMALE STERILIZATION
TUBAL INTERRUPTION

D & C
DILATION & CURETTAGE

HYSTERECTOMY
ABDOMINAL HYSTERECTOMY, COMPLETE HYSTERECTOMY

HIP FRACTURE
OPEN REDUCTION OF FRACTURE OF THE HIP

KNEE JOINT
ARTHROPLASTY

KNEE CARTILAGE
ARTHROSCOPY, EXCISION OF SEMILUNAR CARTILAGE OF THE KNEE

FOREARM FRACTURE
OPEN REDUCTION OF FRACTURE OF THE FOREARM

BUNION REMOVAL
BUNIONECTOMY

*Cardiac catheterization was first attempted by **Werner Forssman**, a young German doctor in 1929. He was convinced the procedure was possible but his superiors disagreed. To prove them wrong, Forssman made an incision in his arm and inserted a rubber tube 24 inches until it entered his heart. He walked unaided through the hospital corridors until he reached the x-ray room and demanded x-rays be taken to prove that the catheter had indeed entered his heart. During the next 2 years Forssman performed the experiment 8 times, once even performing a primitive angiogram—and all the while he was ridiculed by his colleagues. In 1956, years after he had given up his experimentation and moved to a small town where he practiced as a surgeon, Forssman received word that he would share the Nobel Prize for Medicine for his pioneering exploration of the inner recesses of the heart.*

Surgical sponges, made of cotton, gauze or absorbable gelatin, are used to control bleeding during surgery. One member of the surgical team is responsible for counting the sponges before and after surgery to make sure that none have been left inside the patient's body.

*The **renunculus** flower on the cover of this book is particularly high in vitamin C. Its juices were once applied to warts and its young leaves were eaten to prevent scurvy.*

---

2. **Spinal anesthetic** is administered through an injection into the spinal canal. You are awake, though sometimes another drug is used to make you relax or become sleepy. Your view of the operation is generally blocked because most people do not want to witness their own surgery.
3. **Local anesthetic** is injected directly into the tissues at the site of the incision so that only a small area involved in the operation is made insensitive. It is usually used for minor procedures, with people who are at high risk for general anesthesia or when patient cooperation is required.
4. **Regional anesthetic**, also called *nerve block*, is injected into the nerves that transmit pain sensations to a particular area, which enables a larger area to be made numb than with a local anesthetic.

Monitoring during surgery.
If the operation involves a general anesthetic or a regional nerve block, your heart, pulse, respiration rates and blood pressure are monitored during surgery. Any blood loss is closely estimated and recorded. If the surgical blood loss exceeds an acceptable level (usually specified as around 300 cubic centimeters in an adult with a normal preoperative hemoglobin level), you will receive a transfusion of previously cross matched blood. The amounts of any intravenous fluids or blood given during the operation are measured and recorded in the anesthesiologist's report.

If you are undergoing surgery with a local anesthetic, you will be constantly observed by the members of the surgical team for any signs of distress.

Postoperative monitoring and care.
Surgery is being performed more frequently on an outpatient or *one-day* basis. Many operations are now performed with local, rather than general anesthesia, a factor that significantly reduces the recovery period and facilitates outpatient and one-day surgery.

After very short surgical procedures performed under local anesthetic, you usually will not require a long recovery period with intensive monitoring.

However, you will be closely observed until you are considered *stabilized* (your body functions are steady). After local anesthetic, patients are usually transferred from the operating room to an outpatient recovery area, where they may remain for periods of 30 minutes to several hours. If you have had a general anesthetic, you will be transferred from the operating room to a surgical recovery room and attended by specially trained nurses. Your pulse and respiration rate will be recorded every 15 minutes during the first hour. The blood pressure cuff is left in place and your pressure is recorded 2 or 3 times during this period.

The postoperative care plan usually calls for pulse and respiration rate to be recorded every 30 minutes during the next hour. If blood pressure has stabilized within your range, the cuff is removed. When your vital signs (heart, pulse and respiration rate) and your blood pressure are stable, a physician signs an order discharging you from the recovery room. You are transferred to your own room or to a surgical special care unit. For inpatient care, the recovery room stay can range from half an hour to 3 or 4 hours.

People with pre-existing health problems such as hypertension, heart trouble, diabetes, renal impairment or any form of respiratory trouble can expect to spend more time in the recovery room than someone without any chronic medical problems.

Length of Hospital Stay

The length of time you spend in the hospital will vary with your general physical condition and your age. In general, people over 65 tend to have longer hospital stays than do younger patients for the same illness or operation. However, the added stay may be as little as 1 day. The over-65 patient whose preoperative general condition is poor may need a significantly longer period of recuperation.

Discomfort and Pain

Individual perceptions of pain vary widely. One effect of many modern anesthetic agents is to block any recollection of pain from your memory. Is it pain if you don't remember feeling it? Another dimension that affects the evaluation of pain is the duration of the sensation. You may experience a severe pain that leaves you seeing stars for less than half a second, or a moderate pain over 24 hours. Who, other than you yourself, is to say which sensation was worse?

Physicians and nurses tend to apply the euphemism *discomfort* to sensations that most of us would call downright painful. They hardly ever acknowledge that anything might actually hurt. However, nearly everybody can agree that some things, such as that tiny lancet used in drawing blood from the finger, cause sensations that we could do without. During your recovery period, oral pain medication will be prescribed as needed (PRN). Check with your physician and nurses if you have any questions.

For each operation listed, we have attempted to describe the usual hospital course that you can expect. However, there may be wide variations, none of which necessarily indicate differences in the quality of care. Sometimes the time when a particular test is ordered or performed depends less on your clinical status than on a resident's case load or the laboratory's work load on that shift. Many variations depend on your general health and fitness. If you have questions about your care, ask your physician.

FACE NERVE

RHIZOTOMY, CUTTING OF THE TRIGEMINAL NERVE

101,000	2-3 hrs	recovery room 1-3 hrs walking and sitting in chair 1st postop day	wear turban-style dressing until incision heals	heavy lifting and strenuous exercise after several weeks hair regrows
Frequency in 1982	Duration of Operation			

Nature of problem.

Trigeminal neuralgia, or *tic douloureux*, is a condition in which intense shooting or stabbing pain occurs on one side of the face. In the early stage, the episodes last no more than 1 or 2 minutes, with pain-free periods lasting for months. Later, the pain-free intervals become shorter. The pain follows the path of 1 of the cranial nerves; however, the cause of the condition remains unknown. The elective surgery to cut the nerve, **rhizotomy**, will bring relief.

Frequency. Just under 70 percent of all patients are women. Slightly less than half of all patients are between the ages of 45 and 64.

Surgical preparation.

The diagnosis can usually be made on the basis of your symptoms, together with the absence of any other demonstrable cause of the pain, such as a recent head injury or the presence of a tumor. To confirm the diagnosis, you may undergo a **Cat scan** of the head or a nuclear scan of the brain to determine if a tumor is present.

In conjunction with hospital admission, you may also undergo the following tests: **Complete blood count, SMA, Urinalysis, Chest x-ray** and **EKG.**

When you are admitted to the hospital, you will be examined by a physician. Because the doctor will pay special attention to the *neurological* aspects of the exam, he or she will assess the function of each of your *cranial nerves*. You will be asked to smile, show your teeth, wrinkle your forehead, etc. About an hour before surgery, you will be given a sedative by injection. You will put on a surgical gown and socks, and an intravenous line will be started in your hand or forearm. The area near the incision will be shaved.

Anesthetic. You will receive a general gas anesthetic, preceded by an intravenous anesthetic.

Procedure.

1 The surgeon makes a diagonal incision running from a point in front of the top of the ear to just near the crown and above the ear.

2 A small hinge-like flap of bone and *dura* (the covering of the brain) is cut to temporarily expose the operative site. An operating microscope is used to identify the *trigeminal ganglion*, a bundle of nerves which transmits information between the brain and 3 areas of the face.

3 The *rootlets* (connectors of the sensory nerve to the ganglion) are cut.

- skull
- dura
- trigeminal ganglion
- sensory nerve

Stages of recovery.

You remain in the recovery room 1 to 3 hours. On the first postoperative day, you will probably be allowed to sit in a chair.

Limitations. You will have to wear a rather flamboyant, turban-style dressing until your incision has healed. It will take time for your hair to regrow.

Drugs. You will be given oral painkiller to relieve discomfort at the point where the hinge-like flap was created.

Complications. Complications are rare following this surgery; however there is the possibility that a small **hematoma** will form in the line of the closed incision.

Scar. The operation will leave you with a short diagonal scar from just in front of the ear to a point above the ear on the side of the head near the crown. As your hair grows back, the scar will be all but totally obscured.

The flap of bone and dura is then replaced over the site and the skin is sutured.

CATARACT REMOVAL

REMOVAL OF CATARACT WITH IMPLANTATION OF LENS

512,000	1 hr	5-8 hrs in outpatient recovery	walking when leaving the hospital, same day	stay out of bright light several wks	strenuous activity several wks
Frequency in 1983	Duration of Operation				

Nature of problem.

When the *lens* in the eye has become so thick that it interferes with vision, it is removed. The thickened opaque lens is called a *cataract*. In order to restore normal or near-normal vision, the cataract can be replaced at the same time with an acrylic lens that has been ground to the appropriate prescription. The most common type of cataract is associated with aging. However, congenital cataracts are found in infants, and diabetics sometimes develop cataracts at an early age. Cataract surgery is elective.

Frequency. More than 60 percent of the patients are women. The higher rate for women is related to the fact that women tend to live longer than men, and most cataract operations in the US, over 75 percent, occur in people over 65 years old.

About 70 percent of the operations performed to remove a cataract result in the implantation of an intraocular lens. Other forms of treatment to restore vision include thick eyeglasses or contact lenses.

Surgical preparation.

A diagnosis is made by an ophthalmologist based on the results of a **Vision acuity test** and a physical exam. Routine tests, such as **Complete blood count, Urinalysis** and **Blood clotting** can be carried out on an outpatient basis, before the day of surgery. Cataract surgery is often done on an outpatient (1-day surgery) basis. The immediate preoperative preparations, such as the administration of a sedative about an hour before surgery, take only from 20 to 30 minutes.

Anesthetic. You will receive a local anesthetic by injection.

Stages of recovery.

You will be taken to the outpatient recovery area, where you will remain for 5 to 8 hours before being discharged.

Scar. There will be no visible scar.

Drugs. After the operation, exposure to bright light may be painful; however, oral medication can provide relief.

Procedure.

1 Although some patients still receive a general anesthetic, most cataract operations are done under local anesthesia. The eye is anesthetized with *topical* (surface) application of drops. Atropine or a similar drug is used to dilate the pupil, and the surgeon administers a local nerve block.

2 The eyelids are held wide-open with a small frame-like retractor. A suture connecting the *sclera* (outer covering of the eye) to a muscle prevents the eye from moving during the operation. Untied sutures, which will be used to close the incision after the operation, are preplaced on the sclera, a safety measure which keeps the operation as brief as possible.

3 A semicircular incision through the eyelid and the exposed surface of the *conjunctiva* (tissue lining of the sclera), exposes the lens. The site is irrigated with an enzyme solution to dissolve the lens ligaments and the lens is lifted out intact. Alternatively, the surgeon may use ultrasound to dissolve the lens tissue with soundwaves.

4 Any remnants of the lens are removed prior to placement of the new acrylic lens, which has been ground to the appropriate prescription.

5 The incisions are closed by tying the previously placed sutures. Suture material is absorbed by the tissues and does not have to be removed.

Labels: sclera, lens, pupil, conjunctiva, eyelid

Limitations. You will be walking by the time you leave the hospital. Your doctor will instruct you to avoid all strenuous exercise (jogging, lifting, etc.) for several weeks, and to stay out of bright light, either sunlight or artificial light. You may be advised to wear dark glasses, both indoors and out, for a week to 10 days.

You will be instructed to clean your eye and apply fresh dressings 2 or 3 times daily. To prevent scratching or irritation of the eye, you will probably be told to sleep with a protective eye shield until healing is well advanced. **Complications.** Possible postoperative problems include: **dislocation of lens implant**, which would require your surgeon to reposition the lens; **infection**, which can be treated with an antibiotic; **wound separation**, requiring your surgeon to resuture the opening in the sclera; and **flat anterior chamber of the eye**, which may resolve itself without intervention in 4 to 7 days. If not, the wound is resutured in the operating room.

The first intraocular lens made of Plexiglas was implanted in 1947 by Dr. Harold Ridey in Britain.

EYELID ALTERATION

BLEPHAROPLASTY

55,000	1½-2 hrs	4-6 hrs recovery room discharged same day stitches removed 3-5 days	discoloration of eyes 1-2 wks	strenuous exercise 2 wks
Frequency in 1982	Duration of Operation			

Nature of problem.

The skin of the upper and lower eyelids tends to become loose and baggy with age. The source of puffiness is usually the *herniation* of fat pads, which can be removed, along with excess sagging skin.

Frequency. Reliable data on the sex and age distribution of blepharoplasty operations is not available. A **Face lift** (rhytidectomy) is usually accompanied by eyelid repair, but some patients have just their eyelids done. Many of these operations are conducted at outpatient surgery facilities. However, in some parts of the country, the operation is done in a doctor's office. Data indicates that 85 percent of all patients were women over the age of 35.

Surgical preparation.

Your plastic surgeon will take close-up photographs of your face and may ask you to write a brief description of the results you hope to obtain. If you wear contact lenses, be sure to remove them before surgery. You should plan to wear your glasses during the postoperative healing period.

Anesthetic. Many surgeons use a local injection anesthetic for this operation. However, some prefer an intravenous general anesthetic.

Stages of recovery.

You will be taken to the outpatient recovery room, where you will be checked for any evidence of bleeding or sedative aftereffects. When your condition has *stabilized*, you will be sent home. Your surgeon and the hospital usually insist that you are accompanied by a relative or friend. Stitches will be removed in the doctor's office between the third and fifth postoperative days.

Procedure.

1 The surgeon marks the incision lines before beginning the operation. In the upper lid, the cut is made in the crease where the skin normally folds when the eye is open. The extra eyelid skin is cut away, along with extra fat pad tissue. Only the amount necessary to retain proper closing of the eyelid is left. The skin and subcutaneous tissue are sewn closed.

2 For the lower lid, the cut is made just below the eyelash line. At the outer edge of the eye, the cut is slanted upward into a laugh line. Gentle pressure is placed on the eyeball and the bulging fat pads and extra skin are trimmed. The skin and subcutaneous tissue are sewn closed.

3 The eyelids are coated with an antibiotic ointment, and if the surgeon prefers, a dressing is placed over the incisions.

Limitations. Your surgeon will instruct you to avoid all heavy lifting and strenuous exercise for at least a couple of weeks. Of course, you must treat your face gently when washing or applying makeup. You may want to wear sunglasses until your stitches fade. Because the little *capillaries* around the eyes drain into the area below the lower lid, you will have some discoloration under your eyes, similar to a black eye. This discoloration can be hidden by makeup.

Drugs. You may be given oral medication for postoperative discomfort.

Complications. Complications following blepharoplasty are extremely rare. If **infection** occurs, you will receive an antibiotic.

Scar. You will have very fine scars. In the upper eyelid, the scar will be hidden in the normal fold line. In the lower lid, it will be concealed in the line that runs below your eyelashes. Although the scars may be rather pink at first, they will fade with time and become practically invisible.

FACE LIFT

RHYTIDECTOMY	**35,000**	**3½–4½ hrs**	go directly to your room / bandages removed / incisions checked next morning	discharged first postop day / first stitches removed 5 days	remaining stitches removed 1-2 wks / swelling disappears 2-3 wks	strenuous exercise 3-4 wks
	Frequency in 1982	Duration of Operation			

Nature of problem.

The skin, subcutaneous tissue and underlying muscles of the lower face and neck sag with age, producing folds and wrinkles. Surgical correction of the effects of age on the face is becoming increasingly common for both sexes.

Rhytidectomy, or face lift, is elective surgery.

Frequency. Ninety percent of all patients are women. Eighty percent of all patients are 45 to 64 years old.

Surgical preparation.

You will be examined in the office of the plastic surgeon. When the decision has been made to schedule the operation, you will be photographed. You may be asked to write a brief statement describing the results you hope for. Before admission to the hospital, you may have the following tests and studies: **Complete blood count, SMA, Urinalysis, Chest x-ray and EKG.**

The American Academy of Facial and Reconstructive Surgery has a toll-free information service that can answer questions for people who are considering facial plastic surgery. Call 800-332-FACE.

You will be admitted to the hospital the morning of the day of your surgery. About an hour before your operation, you will receive a sedative by injection and put on a surgical cap, gown and socks. A needle will be inserted in a vein in the back of one hand, to be connected to an intravenous line in the operating room.

Anesthetic. You will probably have an intravenous general anesthetic.

Stages of recovery.

You probably will be taken directly to your room rather than to the recovery room, because you will be conscious shortly after the administration of the anesthetic is stopped. Most plastic surgeons prefer that you remain in the hospital for 1 night after surgery. The next morning, the surgeon will remove the bandages and drains and examine the incisions. Usually, a nurse helps you rinse your hair before you leave the hospital.

Limitations. You probably will be instructed to remain in bed the first night after surgery, except to go to the bathroom. You will be advised to avoid heavy lifting and all strenuous exercise, including aerobics and running, for 3 or 4 weeks.

Procedure.

1 While on your back, your face, ears and neck are cleansed, and the planned incision is traced with a marker. This starts at the temple, goes down in front of the ear and, then up behind the ear on both sides of the face. Where possible, the surgeon hides the incision behind the hairline.

2 The skin of the lower face is freed up. The next two layers of tissue are pulled upward and back, and extra fat is removed. The outer skin is then redraped and the excess skin is trimmed. The skin flaps are clamped under the skin in front of the ear. The same procedure is performed on the scalp behind the ear.

3 The skin then is closed and fixed into position with tiny sutures. Many surgeons insert drains in the scalp incisions.

4 The entire process is repeated on the other side. The suture lines are covered with an antibiotic-impregnated gauze, and cotton padding is placed around and behind the ears. The head and neck are wrapped in a bulky dressing to place light pressure on the skin flaps. Some surgeons use a neck collar to support the neck and keep it still.

The surgeon will remove the first stitches on about the fifth postoperative day. In the course of 2 or 3 subsequent office visits, he or she will remove the rest. Your lower face will probably be a little swollen for 2 or 3 weeks, but the swelling will gradually disappear.

Drugs. In the course of the operation, the surgeon will inject with a local anesthetic.

Complications. Complications are rare following a face lift. If blood oozed into a suture line, a **hematoma** might form. The hematoma would be aspirated with a needle.

Scar. You will have fine scars. Some of them will be behind your ears or hidden behind your hairline. If the *classic* face lift is done, there will be a pencil-line scar just in front of each ear. The scars in front of and behind the ear, as well as any running along the hairline at the back of the neck, fade rapidly and become practically invisible over the course of a few months.

NOSE JOB

RHINOPLASTY

51,000 Frequency in 1983

2-3 hrs Duration of Operation

recovery room 30-90 minutes with ice bag on your face to prevent swelling

outpatient, discharged same day, inpatient discharged next day discoloration 1-2 wks

strenuous exercise 2 wks

Nature of problem.

Although many *nose jobs* are performed for cosmetic reasons, accidents, fractures and breathing difficulty due to a *deviated septum* (central cartilage pushed to one side or the other) may also necessitate *rhinoplasty*. In general, rhinoplasty is elective surgery.

Frequency. Seventy-five percent of all patients are women; almost eighty percent of all patients are between the ages of 15 and 44.

In the 16th century, Gaspare Tagliozzi developed a technique for facial plastic surgery. His reconstruction of the nose involved cutting a flap of skin from the patient's upper arm. The flap was then attached to the face while the patient's arm was held in a harness, enabling the blood in the arm to keep the skin alive as it grafted to the face. After 14 days, the flap of skin was cut away from the arm, and the nose was bandaged. In another 14 days, Tagliozzi began forming the shapeless skin into a nose. Many of his patients had been injured in duels or had lost part of their face as punishment for a crime.

Surgical preparation.

As part of the evaluation process before making the decision to operate, your plastic surgeon or **ENT** (ear, nose and throat) physician will take x-rays of your nose and *paranasal sinuses*. He or she will photograph frontal and profile views of your face. You may be asked to give a short written or verbal statement expressing your reasons for wanting the operation and a description of your expectations. Before your admission to the hospital, the following studies may be performed: **Complete blood count, SMA, Urinalysis, Chest x-ray, EKG** and **Blood clotting tests.** You will probably be admitted on the day of surgery. An hour before the operation, you will receive a sedative by injection and dress in a surgical cap, gown and socks. An IV will be started.

Anesthetic. You will receive local anesthetic by injection. Your surgeon will repeat this process during the course of the operation, numbing the various structures as he or she works on them. You are almost always awake during the operation and can hear some of what is going on.

Procedure.

1. With instruments inserted through the nostrils, the nasal bones are fractured and then repositioned to achieve the desired shape. Any extra bone or cartilage (flexible connective tissue) is shaved down and removed through the nostrils.

2. Internal packing and an external nasal splint prevent the nose from shifting while it heals.

3. In the outpatient recovery area, the patient remains under observation for several hours.

Stages of recovery.

You will probably remain in the recovery room for 30 minutes to 1 1/2 hours and will probably have an ice bag on your face to control swelling and pain. If you are to be sent home the same day, you will probably remain in the outpatient recovery area for another couple of hours. In some cases you remain in the hospital overnight and leave the next morning.

Limitations. You won't be instantly beautiful following surgery. You may have a couple of terrific shiners. If this happens, the discoloration can be masked with opaque makeup designed for this purpose. Your face will also be swollen, and there will be some discomfort from swelling of nasal tissues. You will be instructed to refrain from any heavy exercise for a couple of weeks.

Drugs. You will be given oral medication for postoperative pain.

Complications. Some **postoperative bleeding** could occur, which is why you remain under observation following surgery. If this happens, the packing in the nasal passages is replaced and an ice bag placed on your face.

Scar. There will be no external scarring.

nasal bones
cartilage
nostril

TONSIL REMOVAL — TONSILLECTOMY

303,000	1–2½ hrs	30–90 minutes on your side in recovery room painkiller for postop pain upon waking from anesthesia	waking 6 hrs	sore throat several days strenuous activity 2 wks
Frequency in 1982	Duration of Operation			

Nature of problem.

A tonsillectomy is performed for these reasons when a patient is over 5 years old: a history of 4 or more documented tonsillitis attacks a year; at least 2 throat cultures positive for **streptococcus bacteria**; severe recurrent **middle ear infection** (*otitis media*) with hearing loss. The adenoids are almost always removed (adenoidectomy), especially if they are very enlarged and block the rear of the nose.

Frequency. Of the tonsillectomies performed in 1982, 89 percent of the patients were under 15 years old.

Before admission to the hospital, you will have these tests and studies: **Complete blood count, Urinalysis, Blood clotting series and Chest x-ray.**

Adenoids, located at the back of the nose, above the tonsils, also help to protect children from respiratory infections. At about age 5, they begin to shrink and virtually disappear by puberty. If they become infected, antibiotics are usually effective. If untreated, the infection can spread to the middle ear. Because the adenoids disappear with time, surgical removal is a last resort. But if the infection occurs in conjunction with tonsillitis, then a tonsilloadenoidectomy (T&A) may

Surgical preparation.

About an hour before surgery, you will receive a tranquilizer injection, change into a surgical gown, cap and socks, and if you are an adult or adolescent, the needle for an intravenous fluid line will be placed in the back of your hand. For a young child, this is delayed until after the anesthesia has been given in the operating room.

Anesthetic. General anesthetic is used for the procedure.

The tonsils, which are part of the immune (lymphatic) system, help protect children from respiratory infections. They are very small at birth, gradually reaching their full size by age 6 or 7. As a child grows older, the tonsils tend to shrink. However, the tonsils may become infected from a virus or bacteria causing them to become unusually large, and you may be able to see pus and white spots on them. This condition, tonsillitis, is often accompanied by fever, pain in the throat, tenderness in the neck and a cough; it is first treated with antibiotics. However, if a child has recurrent tonsillitis or the infection interferes with general health, breathing or hearing, your physician may advise removing the tonsils. This is only used as a last resort, contrary to the common myth that all children should have their tonsils removed.

Procedure.

1 You are placed on your back, with your head tilted slightly backward.

2 The *mucosa* (soft, moist tissue lining the throat) is opened to reveal the tonsil. The surgeon slowly dissects or teases the tonsil and its encasing tissue away from the *fossa* (muscle bed). Extensive cutting of the *mucosa* is carefully avoided.

3 The tonsil is now connected to the throat only at its base. A snare (a thin wire loop) is slowly tightened around the base, freeing the entire tonsil from the throat. This procedure is repeated for the second tonsil on the other side of the throat. The tonsils may be sent to the pathology laboratory for analysis.

Stages of recovery.

Immediately following your operation, you will be positioned on your side with your mouth pointing slightly downward. The foot of your bed will be raised a little above your head, to prevent blood and mucus from flowing downward into your lungs. This also helps in early detection of any bleeding. You will be in the recovery room for 30 to 90 minutes, while being closely watched for bleeding and any difficulty breathing.

As soon as you begin to wake from the anesthesia, you will be given a pain-killer by injection.

Your throat will be sore for several days and you will have difficulty swallowing. Ice cream is a welcome and favorite treatment.

Limitations. Strenuous activity should be avoided for a couple of weeks.

Drugs. You will be given an oral medicine for your throat pain.

Complications. Other than a sore throat and difficulty swallowing for the first few days after surgery, there are usually no complications.

PACEMAKER
PERMANENT CARDIAC PACEMAKER IMPLANTATION

130,000 Frequency in 1982

45-90 min Duration of Operation

recovery room 1-2 hrs | EKG within 24 hrs | walk during telemetry monitoring | strenuous activity several wks

Nature of problem.

The tissues of your heart contain 3 types of specialized cells that make your heart beat. They are called *pacemaker cells*. Heart rhythm disorders occur when 1 or more of these 3 types of cells malfunction (the most common of which is known as *sick sinus syndrome*), or when the impulses from the cells are prevented from reaching the ventricles (*heart block*). Sick sinus syndrome and heart block are the 2 most frequent reasons for pacemaker implantation. Although pacemaker implantation can be planned and scheduled, it is usually defined as urgent surgery. When a life-threatening rhythm disturbance exists, it is performed as emergency surgery.

Frequency. Just over half the recipients are men. Over 75 percent of the recipients are over 65.

Surgical preparation.

Several tests will probably be performed as part of the presurgical workup including an **EKG, Chest x-ray, Complete blood count, Cardiac enzyme levels, Blood electrolyte levels, Blood clotting tests, SMA** and **Urinalysis**. About an hour before surgery, all standard preparations will be made. If necessary, your neck and chest will be shaved. If you have a temporary pacemaker, the site of the electrode's insertion will be exposed because it will be removed under fluoroscopy near the end of the operation.

Anesthetic. You will be given a local anesthetic or sedative, by injection, depending on your condition and whether you are receiving the treatment on an inpatient or outpatient basis.

Procedure.

1 An incision is made in the skin to expose the vein in the right upper outer chest wall through which the electrode will be passed, and the vein is opened. The same incision is used to create a small pocket for the pacemaker batteries in the tissues between the skin and muscle.

2 The electrode lead is carefully threaded through the vein into the right ventricle. When the electrode has been properly positioned in the tip of the right ventricle, evaluation and testing procedures begin. The doctor uses a fluoroscope, both to guide the electrode to the ventricle and to observe the action of the heart. You will be asked to cough and breathe deeply so that the position and stability of the electrode can be evaluated.

3 When test results meet the requirements, the lead is secured to the muscle with sutures. The lead is then connected to the generator and placed in the skin pocket. X-rays are taken to show the position of the electrode.

This procedure is called the transvenous, or through-the-vein approach, which is used in about 80 percent of all installations. If your doctor is using another approach, it will be described to you.

Stages of recovery.

You will remain in the recovery room or in a cardiac monitoring area for 1 to 2 hours. For at least 2 days after implantation, telemetry **EKG** monitoring of your heart will be conducted. In addition, a **12-lead EKG strip** will be obtained within 24 hours of your surgery.

Limitations. You will be encouraged to walk and gradually resume nonstrenuous activity while your heart is monitored. Check with your physician before you resume driving and strenuous activity. Generators last 5 to 10 years and are changed by replacing the generator only; the electrodes are not replaced. You may be advised to avoid microwave ovens because their electrical field can upset the heart rate. However, newer pacemakers are better insulated.

Drugs. You will be given medication for postoperative pain but the transvenous approach used here is not usually painful.

Complications. Though uncommon, complications may include: **pacemaker malfunction, hematoma, wound infection** or **skin death** at the site of the incision.

Scar. You will have a scar near the collar bone, running out toward the front of the shoulder.

HEART BYPASS
DIRECT REVASCULARIZATION OF THE HEART

100,000	4½-5 hrs			
Frequency in 1982	Duration of Operation	recovery room 1-3 hrs	EKG in 12 hrs	resume nonstrenuous
			telemetry for 48 hrs	exercise 6 wks

Nature of problem.

To continue pumping efficiently, your heart needs a continuous, plentiful supply of blood and oxygen, which is delivered from the lungs by the arteries. If these arteries become narrowed or clogged due to *atherosclerosis* (fatty deposits clinging to the artery lining), the heart muscle, deprived of essential nutrients, dies and is replaced by scar tissue. This process is called *myocardial infarction*. To prevent damage to the heart muscle, doctors can take a length of vein from your leg or abdomen and use it to *bypass* or detour around the clogged or narrowed section of the affected artery or arteries. Bypass surgery is considered an elective procedure, but it often has to be done on an emergency basis.

Frequency. Approximately 4 out of 5 bypass patients were men. Just over two-thirds of all patients were between the ages of 45 and 64.

Surgical preparation.

In arriving at the decision to operate, your physician will have ordered several from among the following tests to help determine the condition of your heart, whether it can be helped by surgery, and whether you are strong enough to withstand the surgery. The tests include: **Chest x-ray, EKG, Echocardiogram, Stress EKG, Cardiac scan, Cardiac enzymes** and **Cardiac catheterization (with angioplasty).**

In conjunction with your actual admission to the hospital, the following routine tests will probably be performed: Complete blood count, SMA, Urinalysis, Chest x-ray, EKG and Blood clotting tests. Your blood will be typed and cross-matched in case a transfusion is necessary.

About an hour before your surgery, you will receive a sedative by injection. You will put on a surgical cap, gown and socks. An IV needle will be inserted in your hand or forearm, which will be connected to an intravenous line in the operating room.

Anesthetic. You will receive a general anesthetic.

Procedure.

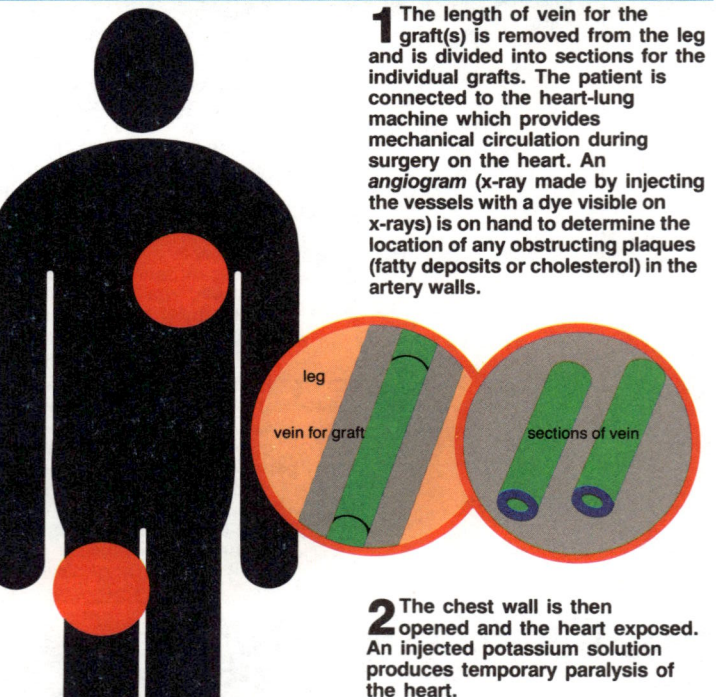

1 The length of vein for the graft(s) is removed from the leg and is divided into sections for the individual grafts. The patient is connected to the heart-lung machine which provides mechanical circulation during surgery on the heart. An *angiogram* (x-ray made by injecting the vessels with a dye visible on x-rays) is on hand to determine the location of any obstructing plaques (fatty deposits or cholesterol) in the artery walls.

leg
vein for graft
sections of vein

2 The chest wall is then opened and the heart exposed. An injected potassium solution produces temporary paralysis of the heart.

Stages of recovery.

Following surgery, you will remain in the ICU 2 days. Your heart action will be monitored by *telemetry* for the first 48 hours after your surgery. An EKG will be performed within the first 12 hours after the operation.

Limitations. You will probably be out of bed and walking within 2 to 3 days. You will be advised to take it easy for 6 weeks and then slowly progress into an exercise program. Most people can eventually return to their full normal activity within reason.

Drugs. You will be given oral medication for relief of postoperative pain, which you will experience both in the chest and in the leg from which the vein was removed.

Complications. Complications after bypass surgery include **temporary disturbances of cardiac rhythm** that can be controlled with medication, and **wound infection**, requiring that the surgical wound be cultured and an antibiotic administered.

Scar. The incision produces a long scar running down from the sternum to a point between the ribs. You will also have a scar on your leg where the vein was removed.

Heart Glossary

aneurysm the wall of an artery or vein becomes weak and bulges out, forming a sac, caused by disease, injury or birth defect.

angina pectoris pain or tightness in the chest that may spread to the left arm and shoulder caused by an insufficient supply of blood to the heart.

arteriosclerosis commonly known as hardening of the arteries, refers to several diseases that cause the artery walls to become thick and lose their elasticity.

atherosclerosis a form of arteriosclerosis where the inner lining of the artery becomes thick due to the build up of fatty deposits (plaque). The artery channel becomes thinner, reducing the flow of blood.

cardiac arrest the heart stops beating and circulation stops.

cerebral thrombosis the formation of a blood clot in a blood vessel supplying or within the brain; 1 form of stroke.

CVA another term for stroke. It may be caused by a clot or hemorrhage that disrupts blood flow to or inside the brain.

congestive heart failure when a weakened heart muscle can not pump sufficient blood and fluid builds up in the lung and the veins leading to the heart putting an even greater strain on the system.

coronary thrombosis a blood clot in one of the arteries leading to the heart muscle, restricting blood supply. Also called **coronary occlusion**.

heart attack in most cases, when people talk about heart attack they are talking about myocardial infarction.

myocardial infarction this is what is commonly called a *heart attack*. When a coronary artery is blocked, blood supply to an area of heart muscle is cut off and that area is damaged or dies. If the affected area is large enough to interfere with the cells that give the heart the signal to beat, the heart may stop beating altogether.

stroke insufficient supply of blood to the brain causing loss of muscle control, usually on 1 side of the body, blurred vision, inability to speak, dizziness, or if severe, death.

Coronary Angioplasty *is a possible alternative to a bypass operation. A narrow tube or catheter is threaded into the diseased artery until it reaches the clogged area. At that point, a tiny balloon at the tip of the catheter is inflated several times. As the balloon expands it flattens out the deposits of plaque (fatty tissue in the artery) against the artery wall, thus widening the channel. The balloon is deflated and the tube is removed. This is most effective for patients with only 1 blocked artery, where the deposit is accessible and not too thick or hard to be compressed.*

3 The affected arteries are freed up enough to permit the surgeon to make an opening below each clogged section. The vein graft is stitched to this opening, serving as a bridge between unclogged segments of the artery system. Occasionally the graft joins 2 points in the same clogged artery, circumventing the blockage. In a multiple bypass operation, 1 length of vein can be used to make several connections, or several lengths can make single connections.

4 When the grafts are completed, the heart's normal pumping is restarted and the patient is taken off the heart-lung machine.

Warning Signs: Heart Attack

1. Uncomfortable pressure or squeezing in the center of the chest causing severe or mild pain that lasts 2 minutes or more.
2. Pain spreading to your shoulders, neck, arms, upper abdomen, jaw or back.
3. Dizziness, fainting, sweating, nausea or shortness of breath.
4. Unconsciousness.
5. Moist, cool, bluish skin.
6. No pulse detectable.
7. No breathing detectable.
8. Dilated pupils.

If you experience any of these symptoms or notice them in someone else, respond by taking the person to the nearest 24-hour ER with cardiac care, call an ambulance or administer CPR if you have been trained. People tend to deny that these symptoms are anything important. If you have any doubts about their cause, take the time to get medical attention.

SPLEEN REMOVAL

SPLENECTOMY

32,000
Frequency in 1982

3-4 hrs
Duration of Operation

recovery room 2-3 hrs | walk first postop day | strenuous activity several wks

Nature of problem.

The spleen is a blood-forming organ that lies behind the ninth, tenth and eleventh ribs in the upper left quadrant of the abdomen. Shaped like a coffee bean, the spleen lies next to the stomach. When the spleen is lacerated or ruptured, as may occur in an automobile accident, uncontrollable hemorrhage results. To stop the bleeding, the spleen must be removed; under these circumstances, a *splenectomy* is emergency surgery. The spleen may also need to be removed for other reasons related to *lymphomas* (cancer of the *lymph nodes*) and with certain *blood diseases*. In these instances, a splenectomy is not an emergency procedure.

Frequency. Almost 60 percent of all patients are men; over 50 percent of all patients are between the ages of 15 and 44.

One of the functions of the spleen is to remove abnormal or worn out red blood cells from circulation. In certain blood diseases, however, the spleen removes the red blood cells too quickly. The normal life of a red blood cell is 120 days.

Surgical preparation.

Your blood will be typed and cross matched. Several units of blood will be reserved for a blood transfusion. Prior to surgery, the usual studies will be performed, including: **Complete blood count**, **Urinalysis**, **SMA**, **Chest x-ray**, **EKG**, **Blood clotting tests** and **Platelet count**. Test specimens will probably be obtained in the emergency room. As soon as the tentative diagnosis of a ruptured spleen has been made, an intravenous needle will be inserted into the back of one hand and an IV will be started to prevent dehydration. Another IV line will be set up, using a vein just above the ankle or in the other arm, which will be used for blood transfusion. You will be given a sedative by injection and dressed in surgical cap, gown and socks.

Anesthetic. You will receive a general anesthetic.

Procedure.

1 After a general anesthetic has been administered, the abdomen is cleansed and prepared for surgery. An incision is made into the abdominal cavity by cutting through the layers of skin, tissue and muscle, which are held open by retractors.

2 The liver, gallbladder, spleen and pancreas are examined for damage. The size and free mobility of your spleen is determined by your surgeon placing one hand between it and the diaphragm.

3 The other organs are moved aside, and the spleen is freed from its surrounding tissues. If necessary, a blood transfusion is administered. Blood loss is controlled by tying blood vessels with gauze packing, and by mopping and suctioning the area.

4 When the spleen has been removed, a portion of the *omentum* (double-fold in the abdominal lining) may be sutured over the remaining raw surface. The area is inspected for any persistent bleeding. The layers of tissue and skin are closed.

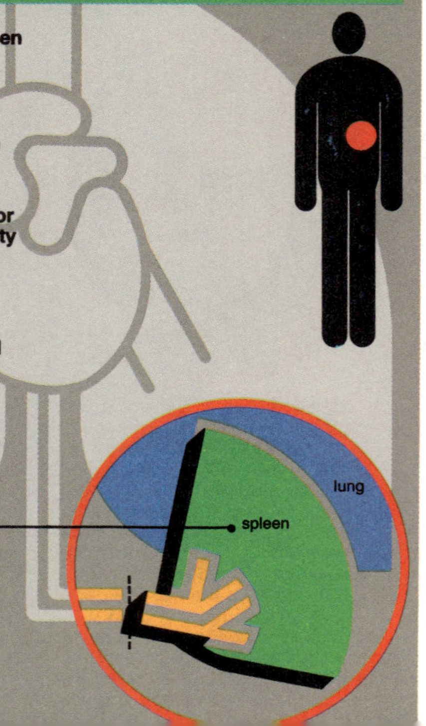

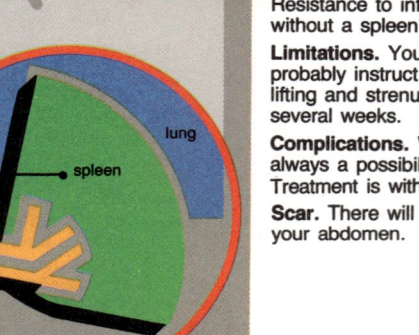

Stages of recovery.

You will probably remain in the recovery room for 2 to 3 hours before being transferred to a hospital room. If a blood transfusion was performed, it will be continued during the immediate postoperative period until your *hemoglobin* level becomes normal. You will be encouraged to walk and sit up on the first postoperative day.

Drugs. You will be given medication to relieve abdominal pain following surgery, and if necessary, something to help you sleep. After 1 or 2 weeks, your doctor will give you an injection of *pneumonia vaccine*. Resistance to infection decreases without a spleen.

Limitations. Your doctor will probably instruct you to avoid heavy lifting and strenuous exercise for several weeks.

Complications. Wound infection is always a possibility after surgery. Treatment is with antibiotics.

Scar. There will be a scar across your abdomen.

GALL BLADDER REMOVAL

CHOLECYSTECTOMY

442,000	1-2 hrs			
Frequency in 1982	Duration of Operation	recovery room 1-3 hrs	walk 1st day	sit in chair 1st day

Nature of problem.

The gallbladder stores and concentrates *bile*, which is manufactured by the liver and used in digestion. Cholecystectomy, surgical removal of the gallbladder, is most often performed when severe inflammation of the gallbladder, *cholecystitis*, occurs or because of *cholelithiasis*, problematic stones in the gallbladder. Gallstones, which may be made of bile, calcium or cholesterol, are fairly common (present in 10 to 20 percent of autopsies) and usually cause no symptoms or illness. However, they can cause *pain, chronic infection* and in some cases, *jaundice*, due to obstruction of the common bile duct. In general, this is elective surgery; however, it may be considered *urgent* due to severe infection or jaundice.

Frequency. Almost 3/4 of all patients are women.

The classic gallbladder attack consists of sharp pain in the upper right abdomen that may radiate through the back and right shoulder. Pain is often more severe after eating and may be accompanied by fever and vomiting. Most cases can be treated with rest, a low-fat diet and antibiotics.

Surgical preparation.

In making the decision to operate, your doctor may have ordered several diagnostic tests that help visualize the gallbladder including **Abdominal ultrasound, Oral cholecystogam** and perhaps **Intravenous cholangiography.** Prior to hospital admission, your presurgery workup will probably consist of **Complete blood count, Blood clotting tests, Urinalysis, Chest x-ray, SMA 16** and **EKG.** About 1 hour before surgery, you will be given a sedative by injection and dress in a surgical cap, gown and socks. An IV needle will be inserted into the back of your hand or forearm for subsequent connection to an intravenous line in the operating room.

Anesthetic. You will receive a general (gas) anesthetic, preceded by an intravenous anesthetic.

Stages of recovery.

You will probably remain in the recovery room from 1 to 3 hours. You will be out of bed, walking to the bathroom and sitting in a chair on your first postoperative day.

Procedure.

1 An operating table with a translucent surface that has x-ray capability is usually used. An opening is made through the layers of fat, connecting tissue and the muscles of the abdominal wall.

2 The *cystic duct*, which connects the gallbladder to the small intestine by way of the *common bile duct*, is cut and *ligated* (tied off).

3 The gallbladder is slowly freed from its *bed*, (the tissue between the gallbladder and the under surface of the liver). This tissue is closed with sutures. The gallbladder is removed and sent to the pathology lab.

4 The gauze packing is removed from the wound. In infected cases, a drain is inserted in the wound, to be withdrawn in 4 or 5 days. The operative field is examined for any active bleeding before closure.

5 The wound is sutured in layers. The skin may be closed with sutures or tiny staples.

Limitations. You will be encouraged to walk, beginning on the second postoperative day. Stair-climbing is usually restricted for a couple of weeks; driving is permitted after 2 weeks. The rate of your recovery depends on your age and fitness.

Drugs. You will be given postoperative medication for pain in the upper abdomen.

Complications. A temporary condition called **paralytic ileus** may occur. In this condition, **peristalsis**, the normal pulsating movement of the small intestine, temporarily stops, resulting in distension (bloating) of the abdomen. The problem usually corrects itself in a day or 2; however, if it persists, the patient is given a bowel stimulating medication. In severe cases, a *nasogastric* tube may be inserted. The condition is relieved when the patient begins passing gas. Cholecystectomy is not considered a high-risk procedure; however, obesity increases the risk of postoperative complications.

Scar. The usual scar is parallel to the rib cage on the right. Occasionally, a midline incision may be used.

APPENDIX REMOVAL

APPENDECTOMY

285,000 Frequency in 1983

45 min-1 hr Duration of Operation

recovery room 1 hr · walk after 6 hrs · leave hospital 2-3 days · drive 1 wk · strenuous exercise after several wks

Nature of problem.

The appendix is a 3- to 6-inch long worm-like structure that projects from the junction of the large and small intestines. If it becomes infected or inflamed, it must be removed. An appendectomy is almost always performed as emergency surgery. **Frequency.** In 1983, 2/3 of all patients were women; 2/3 of all patients were between the ages of 15 and 44.

Appendicitis may develop rapidly with little advance warning. The principal symptom is abdominal pain that begins as vague discomfort around the navel. Over a course of hours the pain becomes much more severe and is felt most acutely in the lower right side of the abdomen, above the appendix. The abdomen may become rigid and very sensitive to pressure. Pain may be accompanied by nausea, vomiting and a slight fever. A diagnosis of appendicitis is usually made quickly and based primarily on an analysis of your symptoms and a physical examination. An abdominal x-ray may be taken when there is time. If there is some confusion about the diagnosis or the symptoms don't seem urgent, diagnosis may be confirmed with blood tests.

Surgical preparation.

Diagnosis, which must often be done rapidly, is typically based on a physical examination and by listening to your symptoms. If there is doubt, or the symptoms don't seem urgent, blood tests and an abdominal x-ray may be performed. Preparations include the usual admission/surgical tests, among them: **Complete blood count**, **Blood clotting tests**, **Urinalysis** and a **Chest x-ray**. You will receive a preoperative sedative by injection, and an intravenous needle will be inserted into the back of your hand or forearm for connection to an IV line in the operating room.

Anesthetic. Because you are arriving at the hospital as an emergency admission, you will be asked how long it has been since you last ate. A general (gas) anesthetic, usually administered for an appendectomy, can only be given on an empty stomach.

First doctor of medicine to receive a degree; architect of the first great stone pyramid.
Imhotep *c. 3000 b.c.*

Procedure.

1 The doctor makes a short incision through the skin and underlying fat. The muscles of the abdominal wall are then separated, revealing the *peritoneum*, the lining of the abdominal cavity. The peritoneum is cut to reveal the *cecum*, the section of the large intestine to which the appendix is attached.

2 After the small intestine has been moved aside, the appendix is carefully freed up from the structures to which it is attached. The surrounding blood vessels are *ligated* (tied off).

3 When freed from surrounding tissues, the base of the appendix is tied off and the appendix is severed. The appendix is sent to the pathology laboratory for examination. The stump of the appendix is inverted into the cecum. The gauze packing is removed, and the intestine is examined. Then the peritoneum, the muscle wall and the skin incision are closed. Closure of the skin will be accomplished with either sutures or tiny staples.

small intestine
cecum
surrounding tissue
appendix

Stages of recovery.

You will remain in the recovery room for about an hour before being returned to your room. You will be up and walking to the bathroom within about 6 hours.

Limitations. Your doctor will instruct you to abstain from running, jogging and heavy lifting for several weeks. You will be permitted to drive after a week or so. Recovery from an appendectomy is generally rapid.

Drugs. You will be given oral medication for postoperative pain in the abdomen.

Complications. Complications are rare following an appendectomy. However, if the appendix ruptures before surgery, *peritonitis*, a potentially life-threatening infection of the lining of the abdominal cavity, may result. Treatment includes intravenous administration of antibiotics.

Scar. You will have a short scar, either diagonal or transverse, at the location of the incision. The diagonal incision, called the *McBurney* incision, is placed in a natural skin fold just above the groin and is very inconspicuous.

COLON SECTION REMOVAL

COLECTOMY

137,000	2-3 hrs		if colostomy, self care instruction 1st day	nonstrenuous activity 2nd day	
Frequency in 1983	Duration of Operation	recovery room 2-3 hrs	begin diet 1st day	walk 2nd day	resume strenuous activity after several wks

Nature of problem.

When a lesion such as a benign or malignant tumor, shows up on x-rays of the large intestine, the lesion must be removed. If it remains, it may become large enough to obstruct the bowel. If it is malignant, it may *metastasize* (spread) to other tissues. In cases of recurrent infection or bleeding, a part of the colon itself may have to be removed.

If your bowel is not obstructed, the operation can be planned and scheduled as elective surgery. If the bowel is obstructed, a life-threatening condition, the surgery is performed on an emergency basis.

Frequency. More than half of the patients were over 65.

Surgical preparation.

Assuming you are not hospitalized for emergency surgery, several tests will be done before the decision to operate is made. These include: **Occult blood** (testing the stool for hidden blood), a **Barium enema** to help identify the lesion on x-rays and perhaps **Sigmoidoscopy** or **Colonoscopy** to visualize it directly. A **Nuclear scan** may also be used to locate the lesion precisely. Routine tests will be performed upon your admission to the hospital. Standard surgery preparations will be made about 1 hour before your operation.

Anesthetic. You will receive general (gas) anesthetic, preceded by an intravenous anesthetic.

Stages of recovery.

Limitations. After the operation, your abdomen will be sore and tender. You will be encouraged to gradually assume your usual nonstrenuous activities. If you do not have a colostomy, defecation may cause muscle soreness in your abdomen during the first few days after surgery.

If you have a colostomy, even a temporary one, you will have to wear an appliance which collects the feces as they leave the stoma (colostomy opening). An *enterostomal therapist* (ET) will show you how to clean the area around your stoma and help you choose a reusable or disposable waste bag. With modern appliances, odor is not a problem.

Before you go home, you, your doctor, the ET and the dietician will develop a diet program that will enable you to eventually follow a regular, predictable evacuation schedule.

Procedure.

1 With the patient lying on his or her back with legs elevated, the surgeon makes a long, vertical incision in the abdomen just slightly off center. The abdomen is examined for any evidence that the lesion has spread.

2 The bowel is freed up from the surrounding tissues, and the segment with the lesion at its center is cut away.

3 The edges of the 2 cut ends of the bowel are sutured together, permitting normal bowel function.

4 If the lesion has caused an obstruction of the bowel, is non-resectable, or if there is perforation of the bowel, a temporary colostomy may be performed. A loop of bowel above the lesion is brought out through an abdominal incision, creating an opening called a *stoma*. This allows the feces to leave the body, bypassing the obstructive lesion. Several weeks later the obstructed segment bowel is removed, and the colostomy is closed.

The surgical wound is closed in layers. The excised section of bowel is sent to the pathology laboratory.

You will have to avoid foods that give you gas, as well as foods such as popcorn, peanuts and coconut that can produce masses that can plug the stoma.

Drugs. You will probably be given a sedative, pain medicine and an antibiotic following your operation.

Scar. You will have a long vertical scar just to the right or left of the middle of your abdomen.

Diverticulosis *refers to the formation of small sac-like protrusions that develop in the lower colon. It is a common symptom of aging and may cause no trouble at all or perhaps occasional cramps, diarrhea or small, hard stools.* **Diverticulitis** *results when 1 or more of the diverticula become inflamed. You may feel severe abdominal pain and nausea.*

Complications include an abscess formation and peritonitis (a dangerous inflammation of the abdominal wall). Treatment involves intravenous feeding to allow the colon to free itself of solid matter, antibiotics and a colectomy, in some cases. A high fiber diet helps reduce the risk of diverticulosis and diverticulitis.

HERNIA REPAIR

HERNIORRHAPHY, REPAIR OF INGUINAL HERNIA

472,000	1-2 hrs
Frequency in 1982	Duration of Operation

recovery room 1-2 hrs | walk within 6 hrs | heavy lifting 6 wks

Nature of problem.

A *hernia* occurs when a small sac of *peritoneal* tissue, which may contain intestine, protrudes through an opening in the muscle of the abdominal wall. An *inguinal hernia* occurs when the sac protrudes downward from the intestine into the inguinal canal, toward (and sometimes into) the scrotum. Eighty percent of all hernias are inguinal hernias, which must be repaired surgically. Women as well as men can get hernias, although they are far more common in males.

The technical name for this operation is *herniorrhaphy*. It is usually performed as elective surgery, in the sense that the problem that justifies the surgery ordinarily is not life-threatening. However, under certain circumstances, the operation may be necessary as an emergency procedure to forestall gangrene of the intestine. This latter situation arises when the sac containing a segment of intestine becomes caught, or *incarcerated*, in the hole in the muscle wall, cutting off circulation to that portion of the intestine. If the incarcerated hernia is not repaired promptly, it can become *strangulated* and may require removal of the herniated part of the bowel.

Surgical preparation.

Upon admission to the hospital, you will probably receive these standard tests: **Complete blood count, Blood clotting tests, SMA** and **Urinalysis.** Your surgeon may order additional studies depending on your condition. About an hour before surgery, you will dress in a surgical cap and gown, receive a sedative by injection and have a needle placed in the back of your hand or in your forearm for later connection to an intravenous line in the operating room. You will also be shaved in the area of your incision.

Anesthetic. You will be given spinal or general anesthetic.

For thousands of years, efforts were made to correct hernias. **Egyptian mummies** *from the third century BC show evidence of surgical attempts to repair these defects. The earliest recorded successful herniorrhaphies were performed by* **Edouardo Bassini** *in Padua, Italy between 1885 and 1890.*

Procedure.

Indirect inguinal hernias account for 60 percent of all hernias. Because they are by far the most common, the procedure for repair of an *indirect inguinal hernia* is described here.

1 An incision is made just above the groin. The tissues are opened to reveal an opening in the muscle covering called the *subcutaneous inguinal ring*, which is the outer opening of the *inguinal canal* that carries the spermatic cord. Here, an incision is made to reveal the spermatic cord and the *hernia sac*, which has protruded through the *abdominal inguinal ring* (interior opening of the canal).

2 The spermatic cord is freed up and held out of the way. The hernial sac is composed of *peritoneum*, the tissue between the muscle and the abdominal organs. The content of the sac, usually a segment of small intestine, is returned to its normal position. The sac itself is *ligated* (tied off) and removed.

3 The abdominal inguinal ring is tightened to normal size, and the incisions in the tissues, muscle and fascia are closed.

Stages of recovery.

Limitations. Your doctor will advise you to do no heavy lifting for at least 6 weeks and no jogging, running or other strenuous exercise for 4 to 6 weeks. Sexual activity is usually too uncomfortable to enjoy for 1 to 2 weeks. Recovery rates are variable because much depends on your preoperative lifestyle, musculature, athletic ability and habits.

Drugs. You will receive oral medication for relief of pain and soreness.

Complications. Possible postoperative problems include the following conditions. **Irritation** and **inflammation of the testis** (*orchitis*) may be treated with application of ice bags to the scrotum, use of a scrotal support, an antibiotic if **infection** is present, anti-inflammatory medications and bed rest, as well as analgesics (pain medication) to relieve the discomfort. **Irritation** and **inflammation of the prostate gland** may be treated by catheterization for relief of **urinary retention**, medication to relieve the discomfort and an antibiotic if infection is present.

Scar. The healed scar is a short, oblique scar just above the groin on the operated side.

BLADDER LESION

TRANSURETHRAL EXCISION OF BLADDER LESION

120,000 Frequency in 1982

½–1½ hr Duration of Operation

recovery room 1-2 hrs

walk first postop day

urinate normally after first few days

heavy lifting after several wks

Nature of problem.

Small localized tumors of the bladder that are not deeply embedded in the bladder wall can be removed with a *resectoscope*. This slender tubular instrument can be inserted through the urethra; with it your doctor can see and remove tissue for analysis and evaluation. This operation is elective, in that within limits, you can choose when to have the procedure done. If a bladder tumor is present, it must be removed and evaluated.

Frequency. Of the reported bladder lesions in 1982, almost 70 percent of patients were men and more than 60 percent were over age 65.

Bladder lesions may be more common in older men because of **stagnated fluid flow** *which may be caused by prostatic disease that come naturally with age.* **Smoking** *is also considered a possible factor.*

Surgical preparation.

Before the decision to operate is made, you may have had several diagnostic tests including **Urinalysis** and **Cystoscopy**, a visual examination of the urethra and bladder through a fiberoptic scope similar to the one used in the operation. **Intravenous pyelography (IVP)** and **Cystography** (x-ray of the bladder) may be ordered as well. Routine testing during admission to the hospital will probably include the following: **Complete blood count, Urinalysis, Urine culture, SMA, Blood clotting tests, Chest x-ray** and **EKG**. You may be admitted to the hospital either the day before or the morning of your surgery.

About an hour before the operation, you will be given a sedative by injection. You will put on a surgical cap, gown and socks. An IV needle will be inserted into the back of your hand or your forearm for later connection to the IV line in the operating room.

Anesthetic. You will receive a spinal or general anesthetic.

Procedure.

1 A resectoscope is inserted through the urethra into the bladder.

2 With a cutting instrument fitted into the resectoscope, the tumor, along with the underlying tissue lining the bladder and muscle, is gradually cut away into fragments that can be passed out through the urethra.

3 The remaining base of the tumor is destroyed by high frequency current conducted by an instrument fitted into the resectoscope.

labels: tumor, bladder, bladder lining, resectoscope, urethra, tumor fragments, high frequency current, base of tumor

Stages of recovery.

You will probably remain in the recovery room for an hour or less. (If you received a general anesthetic, you may remain there a little longer.) On the first postoperative day, you will begin walking.

Limitations. You will be instructed to avoid heavy lifting and strenuous activity for several weeks. In the first few days after surgery, you will feel a constant urge to urinate as the bladder fills. This condition subsides as the lining of your bladder heals.

Drugs. You will be given medication for postoperative pain, as well as an antibiotic to prevent infection. Your doctor may also prescribe medication to help you sleep.

Complications. If postoperative **bleeding** persists or is massive, you will return to the operating room for cystoscopic examination of the bladder. Any bleeding sites will be cauterized.

Scar. You will have no visible scar.

BREAST LESION	EXCISION OF SKIN LESION	680,000 in 1982	10-30 min	recovery room for a few minutes	leave in a few minutes	stitches removed in a few days
SKIN LESION	EXCISION OF BREAST LESION	136,000 in 1982	1-1½ hrs	recovery room =2= hrs	walk 4 hrs	wear support bra 1-2 wks
STOMACH LESION	EXCISION OF STOMACH LESION	30,000 in 1982	**1-3 hrs**	recovery room 1-2 hrs	walk 6 hrs	active exercise after 4 wks
INTESTINAL LESION	REPAIR OF ANAL FISTULA	90,000 in 1982	1 hr	recovery room 1-2 hrs	walk 6 hrs	sit comfortably after 2-3 wks

Nature of problem.–Skin

A small skin lesion (growth) may be removed because it is unsightly, is irritated by clothing or shaving or may be malignant. If it is a flat *keratosis* (wart or mole) or other shallow lesion, your doctor will probably scrape it off the skin, eliminating the need for an incision that requires stitches. If the lesion is *embedded*, such as a *cyst*, an incision is made to remove it. This elective procedure, usually performed in the doctor's office, is described here.

Nature of problem.–Breast

A lump in the breast is usually removed in order to determine if the tissue is cancerous. In some cases, no further surgical treatments are needed if the lump is caught early. Though the surgery is elective, the *biopsy* (surgical removal of tissue to be studied by a pathologist) should be done without delay when cancer is suspected. The procedure is frequently performed on an outpatient basis.

Nature of problem.–Stomach

Common reasons for the removal of a portion of the stomach containing a lesion include *chronic ulcer, simple tumors* that are likely to ulcerate and bleed, and lesions that are possibly

Surgical preparation.–Stomach

To diagnose your medical problem, your doctor will probably order several tests to determine if you are losing blood from a source in the stomach or the intestinal tract and the location of the bleeding source, if any. Some of the tests might include a **Barium swallow**, an **Occult blood** test (detects blood in the stool), an **Upper GI**, computerized **scans** to determine the location of the lesion and **Gastroscopy** to obtain tissue samples for microscopic study and analysis.

If these tests indicate that you need surgery, you will undergo additional routine tests before surgery. For **gastrectomy**, you will be admitted to the hospital the afternoon before surgery. Your orders will include *NPO, nothing by mouth*, after midnight. Your surgeon will also limit your diet to ensure that your food and fluid intake are appropriate. About an hour before surgery, all routine preparations will be made.

Anesthetic. A general anesthetic is usually used for this procedure.

Surgical preparation.–Anal Fistula

Your doctor will probably be able to make a diagnosis based on your reported symptoms and a physical exam. If surgery is considered, you will

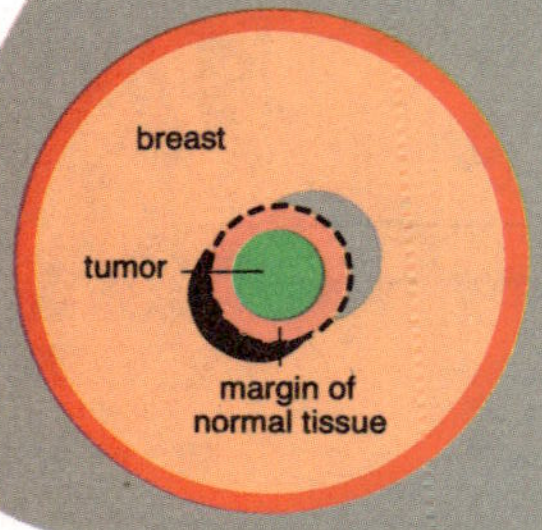

Procedure.

There are two surgical procedures most commonly used in the treatment of gastric or duodenal ulcer. These are the **Billroth I** and **Billroth II** procedures. The Billroth I procedure is described here.

Procedure.

1 The skin and subcutaneous fat are opened. The tumor, along with some of the surrounding normal tissue, is dissected away from the breast tissue and removed.

2 The specimen is sent to the pathology laboratory for microscopic study.

3 The surgical wound is closed in layers and a dressing applied.

breast — tumor — margin of normal tissue

Procedure.

1 The doctor injects a local anesthetic in and around the cleaned operative site. For an embedded skin tumor lesion, such as a small cyst, an incision is made at or near the growth. The lesion, together with a margin of normal tissue, is dissected and removed.

2 The edges of the incision are brought together and sutured. In a facial or neck operation, closely-plated stitches of a very fine suture material are used to minimize scarring.

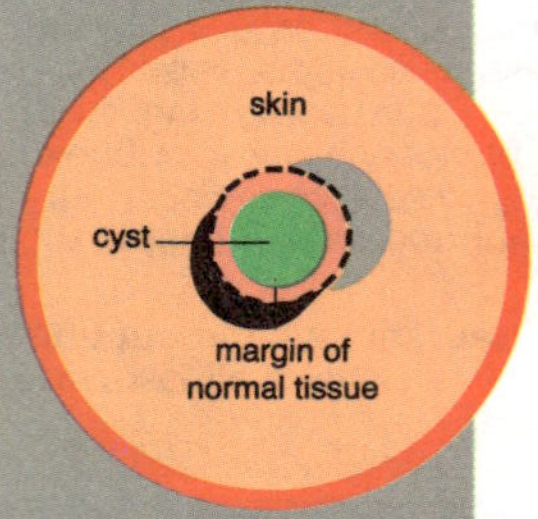

3 The patient is given instructions for after-care. If there are a number of stitches, the

skin — cyst — margin of normal tissue

Limitations. You will probably be advised to avoid strenuous exercise for several weeks, in particular any activity which involves bouncing (such as jogging or aerobics) or raising your arm (such as golf or tennis).

Drugs. Your breast will be sore for at least 10 days. You will be given oral pain medication for relief.

Complications. Infection of the surgical opening is possible but unlikely. It would be treated with an antibiotic.

Scar. You will have a scar depending upon the location of the incision. The most common scar falls on the lower edge of the nipple. Reconstructive or cosmetic surgery is possible.

Stages of recovery.–Stomach

You will probably spend 1 to 2 hours in the recovery room. You may be encouraged to get out of bed to go to the bathroom on the first postoperative day.

Limitations. You will be advised to avoid active exercise for about 4 weeks and heavy lifting for at least 6 weeks. You should ask your physician about diet restrictions.

Drugs. You will receive medication for postoperative pain and an antidiarrheal medication if you experience diarrhea.

precancerous. Removal of a stomach lesion is considered elective surgery. Depending upon the type and severity of the growth, your physician may remove as much as 2/3 of the stomach resulting in a **partial gastrectomy**.

Nature of problem.-Anal Fistula

An *anal fistula* is an abnormal tunnel which connects an internal opening in the rectum just above the anus with an external opening in the skin near the anus. This tunnel tends to become infected, to break down and to need drainage. In most cases, development of an anal fistula follows an abscess in the lower rectum. The only effective long-term treatment is elective surgery to excise the fistula.

Surgical preparation.-Skin

Usually, no diagnostic tests are required. Preoperative preparation consists of cleaning the skin.

Anesthetic. The doctor injects a local anesthetic such as procaine.

Surgical preparation.-Breast

Before deciding to have a biopsy, you will probably have a manual **Breast exam** by your doctor, **Mammography**, and perhaps **Thermography**. Routine tests upon admission include: **Complete blood count, Urinalysis, Chest x-ray** and **EKG** if you are over 40.

Anesthetic. A breast biopsy can be performed under a local anesthetic or an intravenous general anesthetic.

also undergo a **Proctosigmoidoscopy**. Though rare, an anal fistula can be caused by *cancer*, *ulcerative colitis* or *Crohn's disease*; therefore, a **Barium enema** or **Sigmoidoscopy** may be done to rule out these possiblities.

Prior to surgery, you will most likely have a series of routine tests performed. You will probably be admitted on the morning of your scheduled surgery. About an hour before the operation, all standard preparations will be made.

Anesthetic. You will probably receive a spinal anesthetic though a general anesthetic is sometimes used.

Stages of recovery.-Skin

You can usually leave the office or operating room within a few minutes after the dressing has been placed on the operated site. You usually return to the doctor's office to have the stitches removed within a few days.

Limitations. Be careful not to get the wound wet.

Drugs. You may receive a pain medication for soreness.

Complications. If a **wound infection** develops, it will be treated with an antibiotic.

Stages of recovery.-Breast

You will remain in the recovery room 30 minutes to 2 ½ hours. You will be encouraged to walk within 4 hours of surgery. You will probably continue to wear a support bra for 1 to 2 weeks.

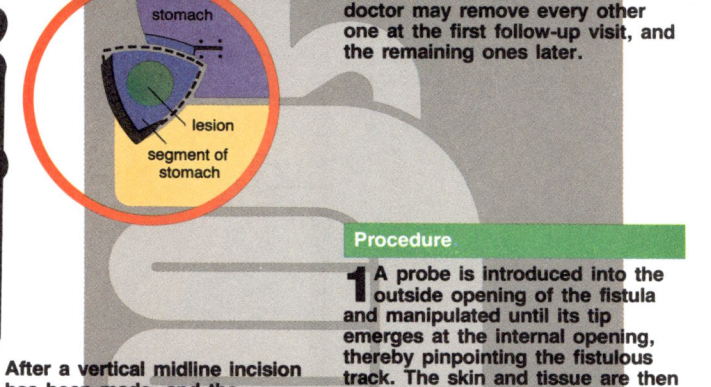

doctor may remove every other one at the first follow-up visit, and the remaining ones later.

Procedure

1 After a vertical midline incision has been made, and the muscles retracted, the peritoneum (lining that holds the abdominal organs) is opened, and separated from the stomach. An opening is made in the stomach wall; the surgeon inserts his finger to determine the exact size and location of the lesion. Suction is used to remove blood from the field.

2 The incision is extended around the lesion, and a wedge-shaped portion of the front and back stomach wall is removed. The edges are brought together with sutures, and the abdominal incision is closed.

Procedure

1 A probe is introduced into the outside opening of the fistula and manipulated until its tip emerges at the internal opening, thereby pinpointing the **fistulous track**. The skin and tissue are then cut open down to the probe.

2 The track is opened and the interior edges of the opening are cut away, leaving a wide wound for good drainage. The wound is not sutured, but heals from its interior up to the surface.

3 A padded dressing is applied.

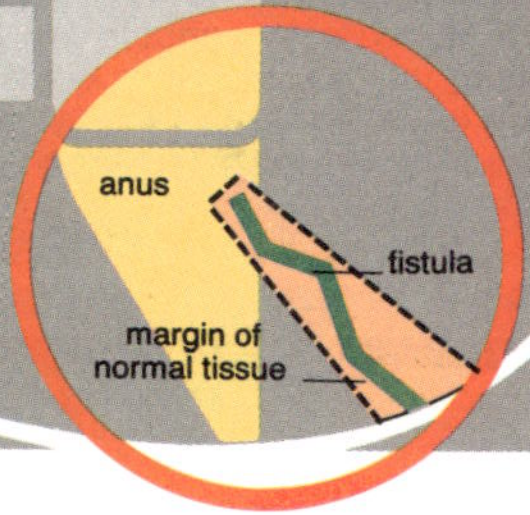

Complications. Complications threatening your welfare do not typically occur. However, some people experience **dumping syndrome** after a partial gastrectomy. Symptoms include excessive perspiration, palpitations and nausea, and they usually occur 1 to 1½ hours after meals. Treatment involves a high protein diet with small, frequent portions of dry foods and fluids between meals.

Scar. You will probably have a vertical scar in the midline or slightly to the right of the midline of the upper abdomen.

Stages of recovery.-Anal Fistula

You will remain in the recovery room about 2 hours and be encouraged to walk within 6 hours of your surgery.

Limitations. In order to prevent infection, scrupulous cleaning will be very important during the healing period. You may find that sitting for long periods will be uncomfortable for 2 to 3 weeks.

Drugs. You will be given oral medication for postoperative pain and probably a stool softener.

Complications. Possible complications include **postoperative bleeding**, treated by suturing the wound, or **infection**, treated with antibiotics.

Scar. The wound is not sewn together. The normal healing process provides new tissue from the internal opening to the outside skin area.

PROSTATE

TRANSURETHRAL RESECTION OF THE PROSTATE (TURP)

| 258,000 Frequency in 1982 | 1-1½ hrs Duration of Operation | recovery room 1-2 hrs | walk 1st postop day | strenuous activity after 6 wks |

Nature of problem.

In men, the prostate gland surrounds the upper part of the urethra as it leaves the bladder. If the gland becomes significantly enlarged, as it often does with age, it may squeeze the bladder outlet interfering with the flow of urine and eventually cause bladder and kidney infection and damage. In TURP, the procedure described here, an instrument is introduced through the urethra and a large portion of the gland is cut away. There is no abdominal incision. When the prostate is above a certain size or cancer is suspected, other surgical procedures (suprapubic, retropubic or perineal) may be used. These are more radical operations where an incision must be made, and a much higher incidence of impotence is associated with them. While TURP is not usually emergency surgery, it may be urgently required to prevent urinary retention and infection.

Frequency. Three-fourths of the men who received TURP in 1983 were age 65 or older.

Surgical preparation.

Before the decision to operate is made, you may undergo several tests including **Intravenous pyelography (IVP)**, **Acid phosphatase** (elevated in prostate cancer) and perhaps **Cystoscopy**. You will also have a group of routine presurgery tests that may include: **Complete blood count**, **Urinalysis, Urine culture, Electrolytes, Chest x-ray** and if you are over 40, an **EKG**. About an hour before surgery you are sedated by injection. An intravenous needle is inserted, usually in the back of your hand for later administration of. IV fluids.

Anesthetic. Usually, a regional nerve block or spinal anesthesia is used.

Stages of recovery.

Limitations. You will be instructed to avoid all strenuous exercise for at least 6 weeks following surgery. Sexual activity can resume in about 4 to 6 weeks when bleeding has stopped and you feel comfortable.

Drugs. You will be given oral medication to control postoperative pain, perhaps antibiotics to prevent infection and stool softeners to reduce strain during bowel movements.

Complications. A 10 percent **impotency** rate has been reported after TURP; however, this may be due to the older age group involved.

Procedure.

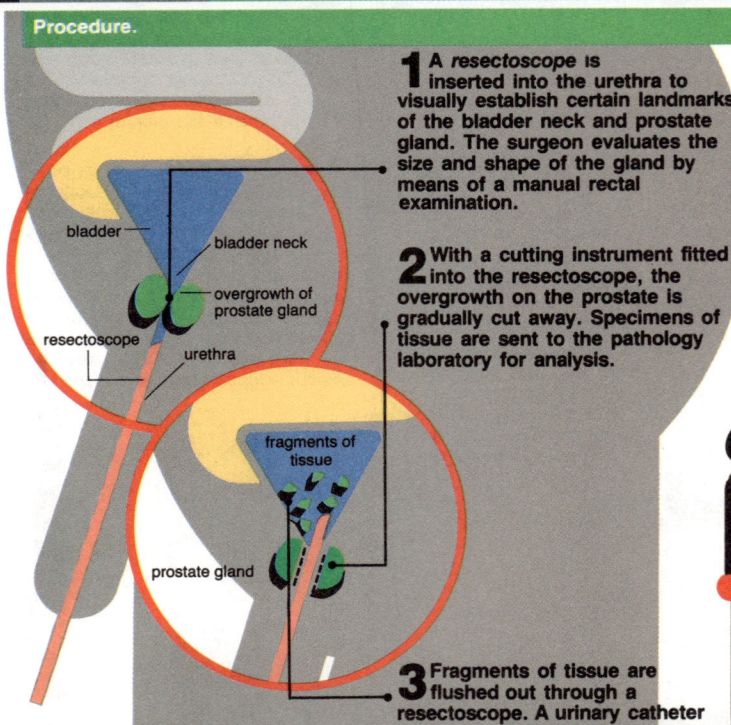

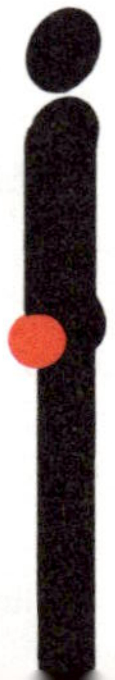

1 A resectoscope is inserted into the urethra to visually establish certain landmarks of the bladder neck and prostate gland. The surgeon evaluates the size and shape of the gland by means of a manual rectal examination.

2 With a cutting instrument fitted into the resectoscope, the overgrowth of the prostate is gradually cut away. Specimens of tissue are sent to the pathology laboratory for analysis.

3 Fragments of tissue are flushed out through a resectoscope. A urinary catheter will be inserted following surgery

labels: bladder, bladder neck, overgrowth of prostate gland, urethra, resectoscope, fragments of tissue, prostate gland

No nerves are severed in the operation that would affect potency. If you had good erections before surgery, you will probably continue to have good erections. After TURP, most patients experience **retrograde ejaculation.** Instead of flowing out of the penis, semen flows into the bladder during orgasm. You may notice the lack of ejaculate, but it is not painful and does not reduce the other feelings of climax. The semen is later eliminated in the urine. **Urinary infection** is another possible complication. It is treated with antibiotics.

Scar. With the TURP procedure, there is no scar because entry is through the urethra, without an incision.

A radical retropubic prostatectomy is a common operation used to remove a cancerous prostate. The incision, which is made in the lower abdomen, tends to injure a nerve bundle linked to erection function. Impotence may be as high as 80-85 percent after surgery. However, a new, nerve-sparing technique has recently been invented by Dr. Patrick Walsh of Johns Hopkins University. Preliminary studies show 60-80 percent of the men who undergo the procedure are able to have intercourse within 6 months of surgery.

FORCEPS DELIVERY

LOW FORCEPS DELIVERY WITH EPISIOTOMY

Frequency in 1982: 622,000

Duration of Operation: 5 min

recovery room 1-2 hrs | walk 1st postop day

Nature of problem.

When labor fails to progress normally and the baby seems stuck, your obstetrician may consider assisting and hastening delivery with an episiotomy (enlarging the vaginal opening by making an incision in the perineum) and use of forceps. This approach to delivery may be considered in the presence of 1 or more of the following conditions: **Baby's head delayed** on the perineum for more than 30 minutes or **second stage of labor exceeding** 1 1/2 hours, **fetal distress** (abnormal fetal heartbeat), **breech presentation** where the baby is backwards and will be born head last, **maternal distress** or **preexisting medical problem** such as heart disease. The procedure may also be advisable in premature births where the infant's head is unable to withstand the pressure of prolonged contractions.

Nearly one-third of female infertility cases involve the fallopian tubes. The tubes may be blocked, scarred or missing.

Infertility has nearly tripled among women aged 20-24 years since 1965.

Every year in the United States, an estimated 8,000 babies are born to women inseminated with donated sperm.

Surgical preparation.

If you have been seeing an obstetrician regularly, you have probably already had a variety of tests including: **Complete blood count** and **Urinalysis**, as well as pelvic measurements and perhaps **Fetal ultrasound** or **Fetal monitoring**. Your blood should also have been typed and cross matched in the unlikely case that a transfusion is needed. During labor, a number of diagnostic observations are made and recorded: the *position of the baby's head* is determined, *his or her heart rate* is measured by a fetal monitor and the *cervix* is observed for dilation. In some hospitals, you are given an enema and your pubic hair is shaved. In preparation for delivery, your thighs and vulva (external opening of the vagina) will be cleansed with antiseptic, with additional antiseptic poured on the vagina.

Anesthesia. You will receive a pudendal block (regional nerve block) or an epidural block.

Procedure.

In some hospitals you are still shaved and given an enema.

1 A **pudendal block** (regional nerve block) or **epidural block** anesthetic is administered. To facilitate delivery of the head, and to prevent tearing of the tissues, an *episiotomy* (incision in the perineum) is made, temporarily enlarging the passage. This incision is not made until the crown of the head is visible.

2 The blades of the forceps are placed along the sides of the fetal head, just in front of the ears. Gentle traction (pulling) is used to deliver the fetal head.

3 Immediately after delivery of the placenta, the cervix and vagina are examined for tears, and any needed repairs are made. The episiotomy incision is closed in layers, with sutures in the muscle and subcutaneous tissue, but not in the skin to allow drainage. No dressings are applied.

fetal head
episiotomy
vagina
cervix
blades of forceps

Stages of recovery.

You will be taken to the obstetrical recovery room for an hour or less. On the first day after delivery you will be encouraged to walk.

Limitations. Your doctor will instruct you to avoid all heavy lifting and strenuous exercise, as well as intercourse, for 6 weeks. You may be given a small cushion or *donut* to make sitting more comfortable while the episiotomy heals.

Drugs. You may receive medication for relief of postpartum pain.

Complications. Breast swelling and pain due to milk congestion may occur after delivery. If you are nursing you will be given hot packs to stimulate milk flow. You may also be encouraged to nurse more frequently. If **phlebitis** (inflammation of a leg vein) occurs, you may receive a blood thinning drug. Your foot will be kept elevated and heat will be administered to the affected leg.

Scar. There may be a small scar which may be initially uncomfortable when intercourse is resumed.

CESAREAN SECTION

Nature of problem.

Vaginal delivery of a baby is not always in the best interest of the health of the mother or infant. Reasons for a cesarean section include: **disproportion** between the size of the mother's pelvis and the size of the infant; **placenta previa**, in which the placenta (the flat, oval, spongy structure through which the infant obtains nourishment) blocks the cervix (the opening through which the child will leave the uterus); **placental abruption**, where the placenta separates prematurely from the uterine wall; **fetal distress**, in which the infant exhibits an abnormal heart rate; **abnormal presentation** of the infant (other than head first); **uterine inertia**, where contractions are weak and ineffective; **umbilical cord displacement**, where the cord is wrapped around the infant's neck; an active case of **genital herpes** in the mother's vagina; or a pre-existing condition such as **pre-eclampsia** (a dangerous rise in blood pressure during pregnancy), also called *toxemia of pregnancy*), severe **cardiac** problems, **diabetes** or other **blood diseases**.

A woman who exhibits none of the above difficulties may be a candidate for a c-section because she has had

LOW CERVICAL CESAREAN SECTION

696,000 Frequency in 1983

½ hr Duration of Operation

recovery room

walk 1st day

Frequency. In private hospitals, 30 to 50 percent of all births are c-sections, while only 20 percent of the births are c-sections in a university hospital.

Surgical preparation.

If you have been seeing an obstetrician regularly, you will already have had some or all of the following tests performed: **Complete blood count**, **Blood clotting tests**, **SMA 12**, **Urinalysis**, test for **Venereal disease**, **Fetal heart rate**, and if you are over 35, an **EKG**. If you are a walk-in patient whose prenatal record is not on file, these studies will be performed at the hospital, time permitting.

Anesthetic. Spinal anesthetic is preferred; however, some cesarean sections are still performed under general anesthesia.

Procedure.

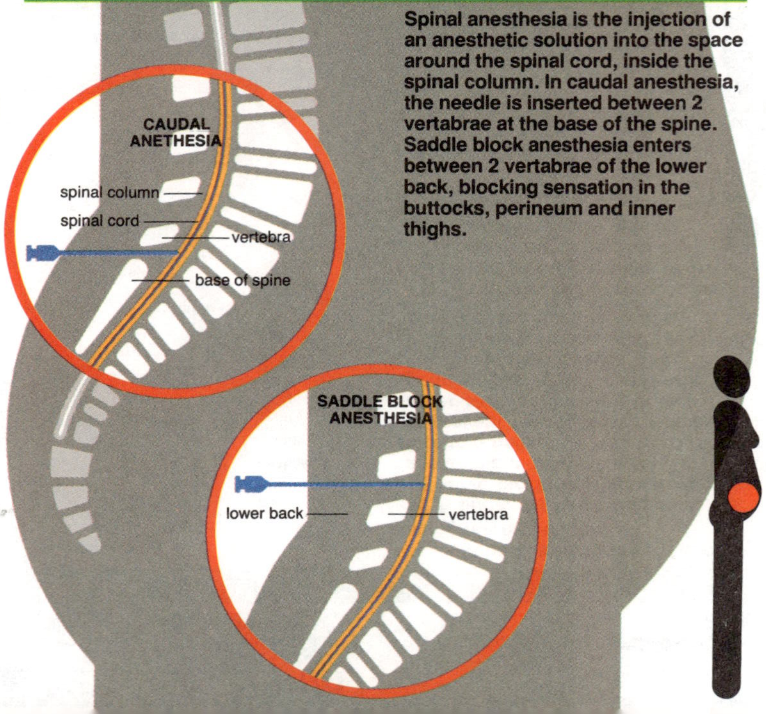

Spinal anesthesia is the injection of an anesthetic solution into the space around the spinal cord, inside the spinal column. In caudal anesthesia, the needle is inserted between 2 vertebrae at the base of the spine. Saddle block anesthesia enters between 2 vertabrae of the lower back, blocking sensation in the buttocks, perineum and inner thighs.

CAUDAL ANETHESIA — spinal column — spinal cord — vertebra — base of spine

SADDLE BLOCK ANESTHESIA — lower back — vertebra

You will be taken to the recovery room, where you will remain 1 to 3 hours. You will be encouraged to get out of bed and walk to the bathroom on the first postoperative day. You may have headaches from the spinal anesthesia. High fluid intake and resting on your back helps ease the pain.

Limitations. You will be permitted to resume driving about 3 weeks after delivery. You will be prohibited from strenuous exercise and heavy lifting for about 6 weeks. Some obstetricians also recommend sexual abstinence for 6 weeks after delivery.

Drugs. You will be given pain medication for soreness in the abdomen and pelvis.

Complications. Breast swelling and **pain** due to milk congestion may occur after a cesarean birth, as it may after vaginal delivery. If you are nursing, you will be given hot packs to stimulate milk flow. You may also be encouraged to nurse more frequently.

Scar. Your scar will depend on the type of incision. The *bikini* scar, a low transverse scar just above the pubic hair, is the most common.

STAGES OF LABOR

First Stage

This is the longest stage of labor and may last up to 16 hours for a woman who is delivering her first child.

1. **Latent phase** begins with contractions lasting 15 to 30 seconds and occurring every 10 to 20 minutes.
2. The amniotic sac may break now or during the next phase.
3. The cervix dilates up to 3 centimeters.
4. **Active phase** begins as the cervix effaces (thins) and dilates from 4 to 7 centimeters.
5. Contractions occur every 3 to 5 minutes and last 45 to 60 seconds.
6. **Transitional phase** occurs when the cervix dilates to 10 centimeters.
7. Contractions occur every 2 minutes for 60 to 70 seconds.

Second Stage

1. Cervix is fully dilated.
2. Duration ranges from a few minutes to 2 hours.
3. Contractions last longer, occur more often and increase in intensity.
4. Fetus descends into the pelvis.
5. Abdominal muscle force combines with uterine contractions to push the baby out.
6. Baby's head rotates as it goes through the birth canal.
7. Baby's head descends to the vaginal opening and the perineum (muscles and tissue between the vagina and anus) bulges.
8. Baby's head appears at the vaginal opening (crowning).
9. Perineal tissue stretches to accommodate the head; if the tissue tears, an episiotomy may need to be performed.
10. Baby's shoulders rotate.
11. Baby's body is delivered.

Third Stage

1. Uterine contractions begin again soon after baby is delivered.
2. Placenta separates from uterine wall as uterus contracts.
3. Placenta is forced out through the vagina and may be accompanied by a gush of blood.
4. Uterus begins to return slowly to its normal size.
5. If an episiotomy was performed, the cut is sutured.

Fourth Stage

1. Observation of the mother continues as risk of hemorrhage, urinary retention and hypotension increases.
2. Mother begins breast feeding or bottle is given to baby.
3. Family bonding occurs.

---

1 An incision divides the skin, subcutaneous tissues, muscle and *peritoneum* (lining that holds the abdominal and pelvic organs). The peritoneum over the lower segment of the uterus is lifted out and pushed downward, exposing the lowest part of the uterus, just above the cervix. The muscular wall of the uterus is cut, then the interior lining is ruptured, and amniotic fluid is removed by suction.

2 The infant's face is rotated so that it appears in the opening. The head is slowly delivered, with the surgeon's hand exerting pressure at the top of the uterus.

3 At the delivery of the head, an injection of ergotamine may be administered to encourage separation of the placenta from the uterus. The placenta is removed, the wound is cleared of blood to the extent possible, and active bleeding is controlled before suturing begins.

4 The baby is handed to the pediatrician to be examined. The obstetrician sutures the inner and outer walls of the uterus, the peritoneal flap and the layers of the abdominal wall. The final layer of skin may be closed with either sutures or staples. The suture process is the most time-consuming part of the cesarean procedure.

High Risk Pregnancy Factors

1. Mother is over 35 years old
2. Mother is under 16 years old

Mother has a previous history of:

3. heart disease
4. high blood pressure
5. diabetes
6. anemia
7. drug or alcohol abuse
8. obesity
9. cesarean section
10. miscarriage
11. spontaneous abortion
12. stillborn
13. premature live birth

Risk factors occurring during pregnancy:

14. unusual weight gain
15. viral infection
16. uterine bleeding
17. multiple fetuses
18. abnormal fetal heart rate
19. abnormal position (not head first) of baby in womb
20. abnormally slow fetal growth

FEMALE STERILIZATION

TUBAL INTERRUPTION

196,000 Frequency in 1982

1 hr Duration of Operation

walk within 6 hrs

with laparoscopy, leave same day

with Pomeroy, leave next day

strenuous exercise couple wks

Nature of problem.

Tubal interruption or bilateral tubal ligation cuts or blocks the fallopian tubes. Eggs from the ovaries are thus unable to be fertilized by sperm, preventing conception. This elective procedure is performed in response to a woman's request for sterilization.

Frequency. All patients were women of childbearing age.

Surgical preparation.

Prior to hospital admission, you will probably have undergone the following tests: **Pregnancy** (to verify you are not pregnant), **Pap smear, Complete blood count, Urinalysis, Chest x-ray** and **Blood clotting tests.** Your physician will also review your situation and your family planning history with you to make sure you understand all the consequences of sterilization and that the final decision is yours. The operation should be considered irreversible; many doctors will not perform the operation on a young woman who has not had children.

Anesthetic. The anesthetic you receive depends on the procedure. If you are to undergo a *laparotomy* (Pomeroy technique), you are likely to receive a general (gas) anesthetic, preceded by an intravenous anesthetic. If you undergo a *laparoscopic coagulation*, you will probably receive a local anesthetic injected into your abdomen, and an IV may be started as a precaution. Other types of anesthetic, however, are also commonly used.

Stages of recovery.

After surgery, you remain in the recovery room for about half an hour. If you have had the Pomeroy procedure, you will then be returned to your room. You will be walking within 6 hours and probably will be discharged from the hospital the following day.

After the laparoscopic procedure, you will remain in the outpatient recovery area for 2 or 3 hours until your anesthesia has worn off and you are stabilized. You will then be sent home.

Procedure.

There are several methods of tubal interruption. Two of the most common are included here.

Laparotomy (Pomeroy technique)

1 A low transverse incision is made, the muscles are separated and the *peritoneum* (lining that holds the pelvic and abdominal organs) is opened.

2 An absorbable suture material is used to tie a 1-inch loop in each tube. The loop is then cut off. As the cut ends heal and the suture is absorbed, they will separate further. Eventually they will be covered by peritoneal tissue.

3 The area is inspected for active bleeding and the surgical wound is closed.

Laparoscopic coagulation

1 The surgeon administers a general, spinal or local anesthetic. A *laparoscope* (instrument for viewing the pelvic organs) is inserted through a small incision just below the navel. Gas is injected through the laparoscope to fill the pelvic cavity, separating the organs for viewing and surgery.

2 A cauterizing instrument is inserted into the laparoscope, and approximately 3 centimeters of each tube is coagulated and destroyed. The incision is closed.

Limitations. After either procedure, you will be instructed to avoid heavy lifting and strenuous exercise for a couple of weeks.

Drugs. You will be given oral painkillers for postoperative pain. Your lower abdomen will remain sore and tender for 7 to 10 days.

Complications. Though uncommon, possible complications include: **infection**, treated with antibiotics; **hemorrhage**, requiring blood typing, cross matching and clotting tests followed by a transfusion; **pelvic thrombophlebitis** (inflammation of a pelvic vein). If this occurs, you will receive an anticoagulant to prevent the blood from clotting, and an IV.

Scar. After the Pomeroy procedure, you will have a low abdominal transverse scar, the so-called bikini scar. After the laparoscopic procedure, you will have a short low abdominal midline scar, marking the point at which the laparoscope was inserted.

Vasectomy or the surgical interruption of the vas deferens (tube which delivers semen to the ejaculatory duct), is elective surgery to sterilize a man. In the US, it is the leading form (10.5 percent) of male birth control among married couples. In 1983, 450,000 men received a vasectomy.

D&C

DILATION & CURETTAGE

731,000 Frequency in 1983

10 min Duration of Operation

recovery room ½ hour

outpatient leaves next day

inpatient leaves same day

Nature of problem.

Dilation and curettage (D&C) is often performed to evaluate the causes of excessive, repeated bleeding from the uterus, to determine the cause of severe menstrual pain or to determine the reason for a woman's inability to conceive. This elective surgery is also commonly performed after a miscarriage (incomplete spontaneous abortion) to cleanse the uterus of remaining tissue. In the case of a miscarriage, the D&C is *not* itself the abortion; however, D&C is the most common method of voluntary abortion.

Frequency. Seventy percent of the women were 15 to 44 years old.

Endometriosis *is a condition where tissue that normally grows inside the uterus grows abnormally elsewhere. Each month these tissue fragments bleed just like the lining of the uterus does during menstruation. Because the endometrial fragments are embedded in other tissue, the blood can't escape. Blisters form which irritate the surrounding area. Scarring and cysts may result. The condition, which is most common in women between the ages of 30 and 40, may cause bleeding and abdominal pain, particularly during menstruation and intercourse. Severe cases may cause infertility. Endometriosis has been called a career woman's disease because it is more common in childless women and its symptoms tend to improve after a woman has had a child. Diagnosis may be established by D & C and laparoscopy. Treatment may include hormone medication, or removal of the abnormal tissue during laparoscopy.*

Surgical preparation.

The procedure may be done on an inpatient or outpatient basis. Prior to surgery, you will be given a preoperative sedative. An IV may be started prior to the D&C or in the operating room. The vaginal area will also be washed. Preparation takes 30 minutes to an hour. If you have lost a lot of blood, you might receive a preoperative transfusion. The D&C itself, however, does not usually result in significant blood loss.

Anesthesia. You will probably receive a regional nerve block. However, some physicians perform this operation under general anesthetic.

Procedure.

1 The procedure uses a gynecological operating table with stirrups. With the patient in the *lithotomy position* (on your back with knees bent), the doctor passes a series of *dilators* (narrow instruments of increasing thicknesses) into the cervix through the vagina, gradually opening the strongly contracted cervical muscle.

2 When the cervix is sufficiently dilated, the doctor enters the uterus with a curette, a sharp-edged loop used to scrape out the lining of the uterus. Tissue specimens are removed and examined by the doctor. They are then sent to the pathology laboratory for evaluation.

lining of uterus
uterus
cervix
vagina
dilator
curette

3 At the conclusion of the procedure, a nurse will put a perineal pad (sanitary napkin) in place before you are taken to the recovery room.

Stages of recovery.

Limitations. If the procedure has been performed on an inpatient basis, you will be encouraged to walk to the bathroom and resume normal but nonstrenuous activity as soon as you are comfortable doing so. You should also refrain from sexual intercourse and the use of tampons for at least 1 week or until bleeding has stopped.

Drugs. You will be given oral medication for postoperative pain, which may involve severe cramps. You may also be given antibiotics to prevent infection.

Complications. In the rare instance of **piercing** *(perforation)* of the uterine wall by the curette, an emergency hysterectomy may have to be performed.

Scar. There will be no scar.

HYSTERECTOMY
TOTAL ABDOMINAL
COMPLETE ABDOMINAL

Nature of problem.

Hysterectomy (removal of the uterus or womb) may be performed to treat: **uterine prolapse**, or dropped uterus; **carcinoma** (cancer) of the cervix or uterine lining; **abscesses** of the tubes or ovaries; **benign fibroid tumor**, causing *pelvic pain, excessive bleeding* or *pain during sexual intercourse*; **bladder prolapse**, associated with urinary stress incontinence; or severe **endometriosis** (fragments of tissue from the uterine lining which have become transplanted in the pelvic cavity) Hysterectomy is elective.

Surgical preparation.

Any or all of the following tests may be performed before a decision is made to operate: **Pap smear, Colposcopy, Cone biopsy, Hysterosalpingography** and **Laparoscopy** (with biopsy). Routine tests will be performed before admission to the hospital. You may be shaved before the operation.

Anesthetic. You will be given a general anesthetic.

Many states, including California, require the husband's consent for his wife's sterilization.

Hysterectomy is a general word covering a wide range of procedures. The surgical incision can be made inside the vagina or in the abdomen. The amount of tissue removed depends on your specific problem, age and general health. In some cases, only the uterus is removed; in others the uterus, cervix, fallopian tubes and ovaries may be removed. If only the uterus and cervix (or only the uterus) is removed, a vaginal approach may be used. An incision is made just above and around the cervix. This approach may be preferred in cases of *uterine prolapse*, when the patient is *obese*, or in cases of *cervical cancer* that has not spread. In closing the incision, the vagina is slightly shortened, which may cause initial pain during intercourse.

Stages of recovery.

You usually remain in the recovery room for 1 to 3 hours. You may walk around your room the day after your operation. Any nondissolving stitches will be removed after about 6 days. A slight, bloody discharge is not uncommon for several days after surgery.

Limitations. You will be walking without discomfort by the time you leave the hospital. Other activities, depend on your overall health and fitness. You will probably be advised to avoid jogging or running for at least 6 weeks, heavy lifting for at least 8 weeks and sexual activity for about 6 weeks or until vaginal discomfort has disappeared.

After a hysterectomy, you are sterile and no longer have periods. If you are premenopausal and had your fallopian tubes and ovaries removed, you will experience all the symptoms of menopause as your body gets used to different hormone levels. These may include hot flashes and perhaps irritability and depression. If the symptoms are severe, your doctor may prescribe hormone medication. A hysterectomy has no physical effect on your ability to experience sexual pleasure or orgasm.

Drugs. You will be given pain medication after surgery and possibly antibiotics to prevent infection.

Complications. Postoperative complications include: **hematoma**, a collection of blood in the tissues; **pelvic abscess**, which may be opened and drained, followed by antibiotic therapy; **pelvic thrombophlebitis**, inflammation of a vein in the pelvis; and **postoperative hemorrhage.**

Scar. An abdominal hysterectomy, will leave a low transverse *bikini* scar while a vaginal hysterectomy will leave no external scar.

563,000	1-2 hrs	recovery room	walk first day	gradually increase activity after first day	resume strenuous & sexual activity 6 wks	heavy lifting 8 wks
Frequency in 1983	Duration of Operation					

Procedure.

1 The surgeon makes a transverse incision through the skin and subcutaneous tissues, separates the muscles and opens the *peritoneum* (lining that holds the abdominal organs). The surgeon palpates (examines by hand) the contents of the abdominal cavity, including kidneys, liver and other organs.

2 The operating table is tilted so that your head is lower than your feet. This causes the intestines to slide away from the uterus. An assistant holds up the uterus with a grasping instrument enabling the doctor to cut it free from its supporting ligaments and surrounding tissues. The uterine arteries are clamped and ligated. The cervix is dissected from the top of the vagina, and the resultant wound in the vagina is sutured closed.

3 In a *total abdominal* hysterectomy only the uterus and cervix are removed. The fallopian tubes are tied and cut off from the uterus, but they remain in the abdominal cavity.

In a *complete abdominal* hysterectomy, (bilateral salpingo-oophorectomy) the ovaries and fallopian tubes are dissected free from the supporting ligaments, and are removed with the uterus.

4 The surgical opening is closed in layers. The skin is closed with either stitches or staples.

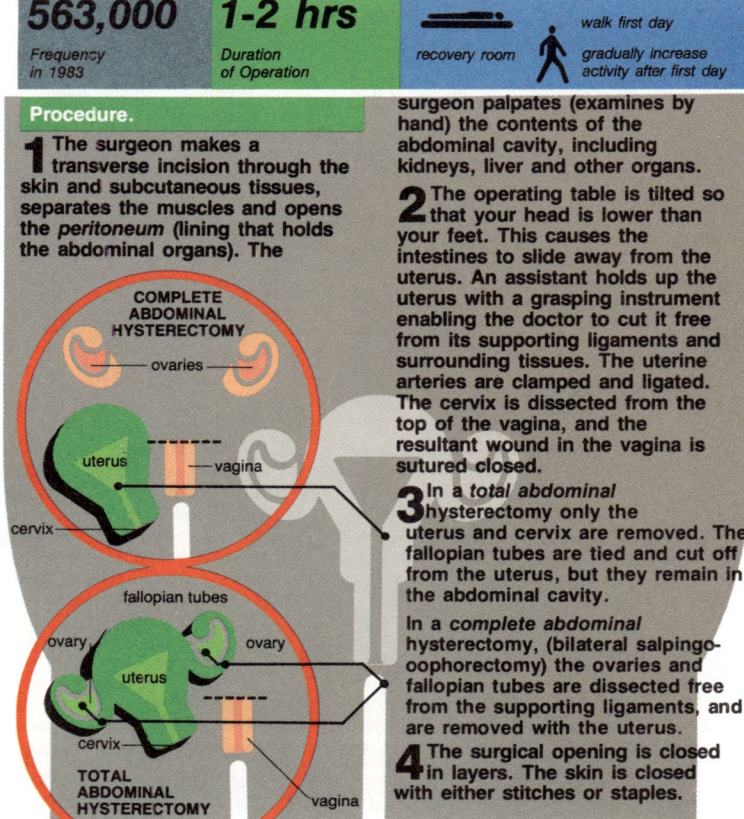

COMPLETE ABDOMINAL HYSTERECTOMY — ovaries, uterus, vagina, cervix

TOTAL ABDOMINAL HYSTERECTOMY — ovary, fallopian tubes, uterus, cervix, vagina

HEMORRHOID REMOVAL

HEMORRHOIDECTOMY

164,000	45-90min			
Frequency in 1982	Duration of Operation	recovery room 1-2 hrs	sit up & walk 1 day	strenuous exercise after several wks

Nature of problem.

Hemorrhoids are varicose veins in the anus. Constant pressure distorts the veins, making them swollen and painful. This pain may be worse if the veins become *thrombosed* (clotted) or *prolapsed* (protruding outside the anus). Drugs, ointments and diet can all help ease the pain and make elimination less difficult. But the most effective long-term solution to the problem is to remove the varicose veins surgically. This surgery, **Hemorrhoidectomy**, is elective.

Frequency. Men and women were patients in almost equal numbers.

Surgical preparation.

Before deciding to operate, your doctor will have manually examined your anus during a physical exam and tested for **Occult blood** (traces of blood in the stool). You may also have a **Barium enema, x-ray** and **Proctoscopy** or **Sigmoidoscopy**, visual examination of the anus and lower bowel with a slender, hollow viewing instrument. These last studies are primarily done to rule out other more dangerous possible causes of pain and bleeding such as tumors or polyps in the large intestine.

Prior to your admission to the hospital for surgery, the following additional studies may be carried out: **Complete blood count, SMA, Chest x-ray, EKG** and **Blood clotting tests.** You will probably be admitted in the morning the day of your surgery, with your operation scheduled toward the late afternoon.

About an hour before surgery, you will receive a sedative by injection. You will put on a surgical cap, gown and socks. A needle will be inserted in a vein in the back of one hand, to be connected to an intravenous line in the operating room.

Anesthetic. Some surgeons inject the tissues with a local anesthetic, while others prefer to have general anesthesia, a regional block or spinal anesthetic administered. Spinal anesthetic is probably the most common.

Your hemorrhoidal stitches will dissolve in 7 to 14 days.

Procedure.

1 Before surgery the anal area is cleansed thoroughly and shaved if necessary. The patient assumes the *lithotomy* position, with knees flexed and feet in stirrups. An anesthetic, either a spinal anesthetic or a local infiltration anesthetic, blocks all nerve endings in the operative site. The final preoperative skin preparations are carried out.

2 One of 2 surgical techniques will be used. Either the doctor will excise the hemorrhoids and tie off their bases, or he or she may choose to excise the hemorrhoids and suture the wounds.

3 A perineal pad is used as a dressing. The patient is taken from the operating room to the recovery room where he or she will be observed closely for evidence of bleeding.

base of hemorrhoid
anus
hemorrhoids

Stages of recovery.

You will remain in the recovery room for 1 or 2 hours. On the first postoperative day, you will be encouraged to sit up and walk about.

Limitations. You will be instructed to avoid heavy lifting, running and strenuous exercise for several weeks.

Drugs. You will be given oral medication for relief of postoperative pain. You will also be given mild oral laxatives, stool softeners and a rectal lubricant to reduce discomfort from bowel movement.

Complications. If early **postoperative bleeding** is massive or persistent, the blood vessel will be sutured. If **postoperative urinary retention** persists, you will be *catheterized*. If you experience a **postoperative headache related to spinal anesthetic**, you will be given extra fluids either orally or intravenously and be instructed to lie flat in bed. You will also receive medication for pain. If the wound becomes **infected**, its drainage would be **cultured** and an antibiotic prescribed. You will also be instructed to take frequent warm sitz baths.

Scar. There will be no visible scarring.

SLIPPED DISC
EXCISION OF INTERVERTEBRAL DISC

287,000 Frequency in 1982

3-4 hrs Duration of Operation

recovery room 1-2 hrs

walk 1st postop day

Nature of problem.

An intervertebral disc (the cushion between 2 bones in your spinal column) is built like a sandwich. It has a tough outer covering called the *annulus fibrosis*, and an inner filling called the *nucleus pulposus*. If the outer layer becomes thinned or injured, the nucleus pulposus may slip out of its covering and bulge into the spinal canal. This is known as a slipped or *herniated* disc, and most commonly occurs between 2 of the *lumbar* (lower back) vertebrae. When this occurs, there is pressure on the roots of the sciatic nerve resulting in sciatica, debilitating pain which runs down the backs of the thighs. When the pain cannot be controlled by other means, elective surgery is undertaken to remove some or all of the herniated disc. Surgery is also considered when pressure on the nerve permanently causes inability of muscles to perform their normal function, i.e., foot drop.

Frequency. Sixty-five percent of all patients were men; 64 percent of all patients were between the ages of 15 and 44.

Surgical preparation.

Before deciding to operate, your doctor has probably ordered regular **x-rays**, and perhaps a **CAT scan** of the spine or **Myelography**, a special x-ray study, where contrast material is injected into the spinal canal. Routine studies before surgery usually include: **Complete blood count, SMA 16, Urinalysis, Blood clotting tests, Chest x-ray** and an **EKG**. Blood will be typed and cross matched in case a transfusion is necessary.

Anesthetic. You will receive a general (gas) anesthetic.

Disc injection or chemonucleolysis is a controversial means of treatment for a herniated disc that may eliminate the need for surgery. A solution containing the same enzyme found in meat tenderizer is injected into the soft central portion of a disc. This part of the disc dissolves and by reducing pressure may greatly ease the pain of sciatica. The procedure, which requires only brief hospitalization, is popular in Europe and Canada where it appears to have a 70 percent success rate. The FDA disallowed the procedure in 1975; however, it has since been reapproved with the use of a drug called chymopapain.

Procedure.

1 With the patient's x-rays on hand, a lengthwise incision is made over the affected vertebrae. After retracting the nerve root at the appropriate level, several of which merge to form the sciatic nerve (the large nerve that transmits information to and from the muscles and skin of the legs), the prolapsed fragment of the disc is removed. Suction is used to remove any additional fragments from inside the disc.

vertebrae — disc
herniation — neural foramen — spinal cord — sciatic nerve

2 When the disc fragments have been removed, the *neural foramen* (bone channel through which the nerves pass) is examined to ensure free passage of the nerve root that connects the sciatic nerve to the spinal cord.

3 The surgical opening is sutured closed in layers.

Stages of recovery.

You will spend from 1 to 3 hours in the recovery room. You will be encouraged to begin walking on the first postoperative day.

Limitations. Strenuous exercise, lifting and running will be forbidden for the first several weeks. Since driving usually increases any lower back pain, you may be unable to drive during this period. After a couple of weeks, your doctor may instruct you to begin a series of rehabilitation exercises to strengthen your abdominal and back muscles.

Drugs. You will receive medication for pain, which may be severe.

Complications. Urinary retention is a possible complication which would be treated by catheter insertion until normal urinary function returns. Any **infection** is treated with antibiotics.

Scar. You will have a back scar where your surgical incision was made.

HIP FRACTURE

OPEN REDUCTION OF FRACTURE OF THE HIP

75,000	3-4 hrs	recovery room 1-2 hrs	range of motion exercises after a few days	walk with walker after several days	physical therapy continues
Frequency in 1982	Duration of Operation				

Nature of problem.

When a fracture of the hip occurs in a person who is mobile (not bedridden or wheelchair bound), the broken bone is usually reinforced with a nail and metal plate. This procedure ensures that the break heals with enough sturdiness to permit the individual to resume walking. If the bones have moved out of their proper alignment in the fracture, the break will first be *reduced*. This means that the bones are manipulated until they are brought back into proper position.

Hip reduction is elective only in that the procedure may be postponed for a day or so after the break. However, it is an urgent condition that demands treatment. Because most hip breaks are the result of a sudden fall or traumatic accident, patients are usually admitted to the hospital on an emergency basis.

Frequency. Two-thirds of all patients were women. More than 80 percent of all patients were over 65.

Surgical preparation.

If you are admitted to the hospital as an emergency patient, the preoperative workup, including **Complete blood count, Urinalysis, Chest x-ray, EKG, Blood clotting tests** and **Blood type and Cross match**, in case a transfusion is needed, is carried out either in the emergency room or after your admission to a room. In addition to the usual tests, your pelvis and legs will also be x-rayed to verify the position of your hip. On the day of your surgery, you will receive a sedative and dress in a surgical cap and gown. An IV will be started in the back of your hand or your forearm.

Anesthetic. General (gas) anesthesia is most commonly used. However, sometimes spinal anesthesia is administered as an alternative.

There are 2 different kinds of hip fractures, requiring different procedures. If necessary, the broken hip is realigned or *reduced* before the fracture is repaired. For realignment, the surgeon flexes the injured hip 90 degrees, then pulls up on the femur while rotating the thigh inward. X-rays are taken to verify the position of the hip before proceeding. Then an incision (4 to 6 inches long) is made in the thigh and the underlying muscle is spread apart.

Procedure.

1 The neck, or top segment, of the *femur* (thigh bone) may be broken just below the rounded, ball-like top of the femur that fits into a socket to create the hip joint. In this operation a nail and a screw are placed through the top of the femur, pinning the neck firmly to the rounded top portion of the bone.

2 In the other case, the break is across the *trochanter*, the uppermost segment of the femur that unites the shaft of the bone with the neck. This kind of fracture is repaired by driving a nail through a supporting plate, and the trochanter into the neck of the femur. The plate extends along the shaft of the femur and is held in place with screws.

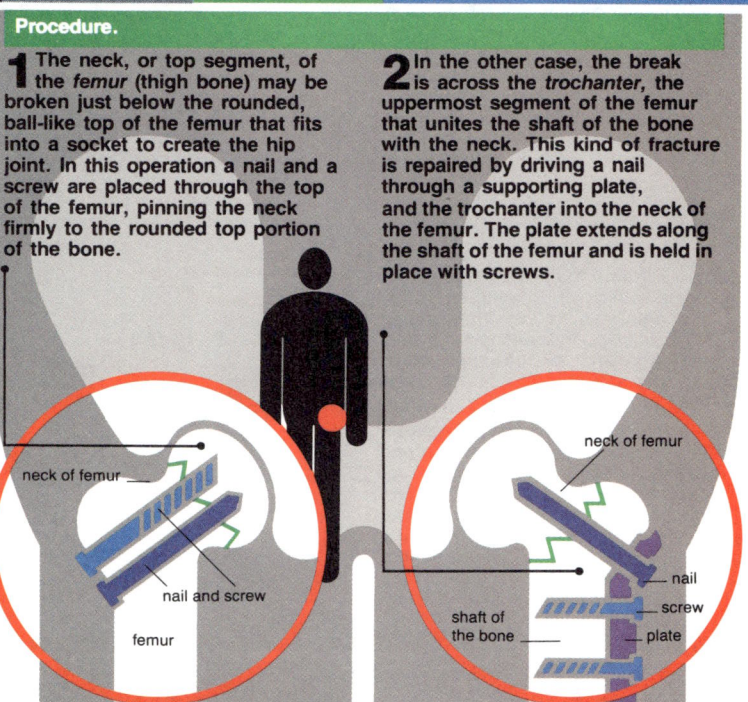

Stages of recovery.

You will spend 1 or 2 hours in the recovery room before returning to your own room. Convalescence is slow after a hip fracture; you will be confined to bed for several days after your surgery. When you are permitted to get out of bed, you will use a walker but will be instructed not to put any weight on the injured leg.

Limitations. Your physician will order a detailed physical therapy plan for you. However, your mobility will be limited for several weeks after surgery.

Drugs. Pain during recovery is considerable. Many patients experience gnawing pain, especially at night. You may be given injections for the first couple of days and then oral medication such as codeine, Demerol or Percodan for several weeks thereafter.

Complications. Possible complications are **infection** and **pulmonary embolism** (blood clot in lungs) which is possible after any long operation followed by enforced bedrest.

Scar. You will have a long scar on your thigh.

KNEE JOINT

ARTHROPLASTY

123,000	2-3 hrs			
Frequency in 1982	Duration of Operation	recovery room 1-2 hrs	motion exercises 2nd postop day	walk with walker 2nd postop day / walk with cane after a wk or 2 / walk without assistance after a while

Nature of problem.

Arthroplasty means *joint building* and refers to the process of rebuilding a damaged joint. Usually the damage has been caused by rheumatoid arthritis or osteoarthritis, which can destroy the smoothness of the joint surfaces. When the problem results in disability or chronic pain, the joint can be surgically reconstructed. Arthroplasty is elective surgery.

Frequency. Almost 60 percent of all patients were 15 to 44 years of age. Almost 2/3 of all patients were men.

Surgical preparation.

Your doctor's decision to operate is based on evaluation of several studies, including **x-rays** of both legs and both knees. Prior to hospital admission, you will probably undergo the usual preoperative workup, including **Complete blood count, Urinalysis, Chest x-ray, EKG, SMA** and **Blood clotting tests.** You will be admitted to the hospital the afternoon before or the morning of your surgery. You will be given a sedative by injection and dressed in a surgical cap, gown and socks. An IV will be started.

Anesthetic. Usually the operation is performed under general (gas) anesthetic. However, in some cases spinal anesthetic is used.

Stages of recovery.

Limitations. After most operations, patients are told to refrain from exercise. Following arthroplasty, however, you *must* exercise and follow the rehabilitation program, which is vital to your recovery.

Your main difficulty will be getting around without putting weight on the operated leg. You will need a walker at first, then graduate to a cane. Your heavily bandaged knee will present logistical problems in showering and dressing. In the early stages of recovery, bulky bandages, as well as drowsiness from painkillers, may limit your ability to drive.

Drugs. You will receive oral medication for postoperative pain, which can be fairly severe.

Complications. Infection of the surgical opening is a remote possibility that is treated with antibiotics.

Scar. You will have a scar from the side of your kneecap to the lower leg.

Procedure.

1 A vertical incision is made from the side of the knee cap to the upper end of the *tibia* (shinbone). The rounded, flaring top of the tibia, the *condyle*, is prepared by carving out and removing a very thin plate of bone. This makes a flat surface on which the prosthesis can be placed.

2 With the knee flexed, the flat prosthesis is inserted into the space between the tibial condyle and the opposing condyle of the *femur* (thigh bone). The knee is then straightened to assess the joint's alignment and stability.

3 The opening is sutured and a suction drain positioned in the wound. An immobilizing dressing is applied, covered by a light cast.

plate of bone
condyle of femur (thigh bone)
Kate prosthesis
condyle of tibia (shin bone)

Arthritis is not so much one specific disease as it is a generic name used to describe over 100 different diseases that affect the joints. They may be caused by infection, or simple wear and tear. (Gout is a form of arthritis where uric acid builds up into crystalline deposits that inflame the joints. Gonorrhea and syphilis can also spread to joints causing a form of arthritis.) However, the 2 most common varieties are rheumatoid arthritis and osteoarthritis.

Osteoarthritis *is primarily caused by simple wear and tear and is most common in the elderly. The weight bearing joints—hips, spine, knee—are most frequently affected. The cartilage that protects the ends of rubbing bones wears away. The underlying bone becomes hard, distorted and painful. There is swelling and stiff limited movement.* **Rheumatoid arthritis** *is more likely to strike people between 35 and 60 and women more than men. It is a chronic inflammation of the synovial membrane, the lubricating membrane that surrounds the joints. Hands and feet are most commonly affected. The membrane becomes inflamed and the joint becomes swollen with excess fluid which scars and damages other parts of the joint. Stiffness, redness and limited movement are common symptoms, and the disease may also be accompanied by a general malaise.*

KNEE CARTILAGE

ARTHROSCOPY, EXCISION OF SEMILUNAR CARTILAGE OF THE KNEE

155,000	1 hr			
Frequency in 1982	Duration of Operation	recovery area 30 min–1 hr	discharged same day	stitches removed 2 wks / physical therapy continues

Nature of problem.

The most highly publicized causes of torn knee cartilage are sports injuries, but the cartilage can be damaged in other strenuous activities, such as ballet dancing. If the pain becomes severe and limits the range of motion in your knee, the damaged cartilage can be removed. It is considered elective surgery.

Frequency. Over 70 percent of all patients are men, mostly between the ages of 15 and 44.

Arthroscopy may also be used as a diagnostic tool. A slender metal tube with a self-contained light source is inserted in a joint (knee, ankle or shoulder) allowing the doctor to detect torn cartilage or tendons and to assess the severity of arthritis. It can be done with local anesthetic in a doctor's office. Some doctors prefer to diagnose knee problems with an **arthrogram**, the knee is numbed with a local anesthetic and then air or contrast dye is injected into the joint. The joint is moved while fluoroscopic pictures (x-ray movies) are taken. The dye helps your doctor distinguish between the small overlapping structures inside the joint that don't show up well on conventional x-rays

Surgical preparation.

Before you are admitted to the hospital, you will have **x-rays** taken of your knee to show any bony abnormalities and possibly an **Arthrogram** which involves a dye injection to view muscle, ligament and cartilage tissue inside the joint. In addition, you will probably have a **Complete blood count, Blood clotting tests,** a **Urinalysis,** and a **Chest x-ray.** If you are over 40, you probably will have an **EKG**.

About an hour before the surgery, you will receive a sedative by injection. You will dress in a surgical cap, gown and socks.

Anesthetic. The surgeon will inject your knee with a local anesthetic.

Procedure.

1 The surgeon makes a short incision over the damaged *meniscus*, the crescent-shaped cartilage on the sides of the knee cap. The incision may be either *lateral* (on the outer side of the joint), or *medial* (inner side), depending on the injury. Through the incision, the physician introduces an arthroscope, permitting him or her to see the extent of the damage.

2 With cutting instruments inserted in the arthroscope, the damaged cartilage is removed.

knee cap
damaged lateral meniscus

View from top
damaged cartilage

3 After closure, heavily padded dressing is applied.

Stages of recovery.

Limitations. Because your knee will remain sore and stiff for some time, you probably won't need to be warned not to run, jump or engage in strenuous exercise or competitive sports for several weeks. Your stitches will be removed after about 2 weeks. Then your doctor probably will have you begin an exercise program to regain strength.

Drugs. There will be some pain, but it usually can be controlled with oral medication.

Complications. There are usually no complications following this procedure.

Scar. You will have a small scar where the incision is made.

There are roughly 65,000 knee implants a year. The new joint alone (not counting installation) cost about $2500 in 1985. Knee and hip joint replacements are made out of the same material used to make fan blades in jet airplanes—a cobalt, molybdenum and chromium alloy that is heated to 2800 degrees Fahrenheit before being poured into a mold.

FOREARM FRACTURE

| OPEN REDUCTION OF FRACTURE OF THE FOREARM | 274,000 Frequency in 1982 | 1-2 hrs Duration of Operation | recovery room 1-2 hrs | hand & arm swell 1st couple of days | walk 1st day | physical therapy starts 7-10 days | arm in sling several wks |

Nature of problem.

If you have broken your arm, and the fractured bones are not normally aligned, it is necessary to perform an operation called an open reduction. In this non-elective surgery, the surgeon brings the fractured ends together in their proper position, and fixes them in place with metal plates held by screws. This enables the bones to knit properly.

Frequency. Both sexes were equally represented with most patients in the 15 to 44 age group.

The bone marrow produces 300 billion blood cells a day, over 3 million a second. In a young person the marrow is a pinkish red. As we grow older the marrow in many bones is gradually infiltrated by fat and turns a grayish yellow.

A recent study reports that hospitalized patients whose rooms had views of trees or parks recovered more quickly than those who had only brick walls to look at. They stayed less time in the hospital, got on better with the nursing staff and requested less pain medication.

Surgical preparation.

Since this is not planned surgery, the diagnostic work is performed after your arrival at the hospital. Several x-rays will be taken to show the location of the breaks and the positions of the bones. Routine lab work may include some or all of the following: **Complete blood count, Urinalysis, EKG, Chest x-ray** and **Blood clotting tests.**

Before surgery, you will be given a tranquilizer by injection. A surgical cap and socks will be put on you and a blanket will be draped over you, in place of the surgical gown. A needle will be inserted in the back of your uninjured hand and connected with an intravenous (IV) line.

Anesthetic. You will receive a general (gas) anesthetic, preceded by an intravenous anesthetic.

Procedure.

1 The arm is placed on a special arm support. A pneumatic tourniquet is applied to maintain a relatively bloodless field.

2 The radius is exposed first, with an incision about 6 inches long, centered over the fracture and running longitudinally down the forearm. The radial fracture is located and reduced (broken ends brought together in proper alignment).

3 A 6-inch incision is made, centered over the ulnar fracture. The broken ends of the ulna are manipulated to reduce the fracture, and a 6-hole plate is applied to immobilize the bone.

4 The radial fracture is again reduced, and a semi-tubular 6-hole plate applied. With the radius fixed, the ulnar plate is screwed in position.

5 Both wounds are closed, with suction drainage to each one. A

Stages of recovery.

Limitations. Having your heavily bandaged arm in a sling will cramp your style for several weeks. It will be more difficult to perform everyday tasks, like showering and getting dressed, not to mention writing or playing the piano. Even after the x-rays show good healing progress and you are fairly comfortable during the day, you may experience more pain at night that interferes with sleep. You may be advised to boost your mineral intake, since good nutrition plays an important part in speeding up the healing process. After a week to 10 days, your doctor will have you begin physical therapy to prevent muscle atrophy.

Drugs. You will receive medication for pain. You may also be given a sleeping pill at night.

Complications. Infection of the surgical opening is a possibility. It is treated with antibiotics.

Scar. You will have 2 parallel 6-inch scars on your forearm.

(diagram labels: ulna, radius, radial fracture, 6 hole plate, ulnar fracture)

BUNION REMOVAL

BUNIONECTOMY

112,000 Frequency in 1982

1-1½ hrs Duration of Operation

recovery room ½ hr | walk with walker in a few hours | walk without assistance 1 wk / discharged next day

Nature of problem.

The *metatarsal* bones in the foot are the long bones to which your toe bones are attached. In most of us, they are straight, but in some people the first metatarsal, which is attached to the big toe, tends to point inward (toward the other foot). This causes the big toe to point outward, so that the head of the metatarsal protrudes. Constant irritation from shoes causes the head of the metatarsal to swell and become painful. This swelling is called a *bunion*. The deformity of the metatarsal is called *hallux valgus*.

Frequency. Eighty-five percent of all patients were women, probably due to high fashion shoes.

Surgical suture material is categorized as either absorbable or nonabsorbable. Nylon and silk, for instance, are nonabsorbable. New synthetic materials and catgut (actually spun from the intestines of cows and sheep) dissolve in the body within a predetermined period of time. Over the centuries, horse hair, moose tendons and gold or silver wire have all been used to stitch wounds shut. The latest advance is surgical staples. They can be quickly applied with a special surgical staple gun and then later removed with a device that looks a lot like your office staple remover. Though surgical staples are used internally, their primary use is in closing the skin where they tend to be less scarring than conventional sutures.

Surgical preparation.

In studying your foot problem, the doctor will have ordered **x-rays** of your feet. Routine pre-surgery tests performed before admission to the hospital may include: **Complete blood count, Urinalysis, SMA, Chest x-ray** and an **EKG**. You are usually admitted to the hospital on the morning of surgery. About an hour before the operation, you will receive a sedative by injection and dress in a surgical cap and gown. An IV will be started with a needle in your hand or forearm.

Anesthetic. You will probably receive intravenous anesthesia.

Procedure.

1 A 2-inch incision is made in the tissue along the first metatarsal joints where the bone of the big toe joins the first metatarsal in the front of the foot. The *lateral sesamoid*, a small bone embedded in the tendons at the joint, is removed and the tendons connected to the joint are cut.

2 The bunion is composed of an enlargement of the metatarsal bone and the *bursa*, a sac of tissue and fluid surrounding the joint. The excess bursa is cut away, and the enlarged bone is chiselled with a surgical saw. The tendons are shortened to realign the altered joint and sutured into place. Where necessary, to stabilize the big toe in proper alignment, small plates and pins are used.

3 The surgical wound is closed. A series of compressive and immobilizing dressings is used during the gradual recovery from the operation.

metatarsal joint
bunion

Stages of recovery.

You will remain in the recovery room from half a hour to 1 1/2 hours depending on how quickly you *stabilize* (when your vital signs return to normal). Within a few hours of surgery, you will be encouraged to begin walking; however, you may need a walker for a week or so, especially if both feet have been operated on. You may leave the hospital later that day or the following day.

Limitations. Your mobility will be impaired during your recovery period. You will be limited to fabric surgical shoes until the dressings are removed.

Drugs. Postoperative pain can be fairly severe. However, you will be given oral medication to control it.

Complications. Wound infection is a distant possibility. Antibiotics would be prescribed.

Scar. You will have a fine scar along the inner side of the big toe and metatarsal joint.

Some surgeons repair only one foot at a session; others repair both. To a great extent, this depends on how severe your condition is.

QUESTIONS & ANSWERS

- CHOOSING A DOCTOR
- WHAT TO DO IF SURGERY HAS BEEN RECOMMENDED
- HOSPITALS
- IN THE HOSPITAL
- PATIENT'S RIGHTS
- RESPONSIBILITIES
- HEALTH INFORMATION
- INSURANCE
- COSTS
- EMERGENCIES

CHOOSING A DOCTOR

1 How do I choose a doctor?

The best time to choose a doctor is when you do not need one. You can then assess your concerns and take the time to interview a few doctors, research their backgrounds and qualifications, evaluate the nature of their practice and then decide on the one with whom you feel the most comfortable.

Check the doctor's prices, fee schedules and whether or not he or she accepts Medicare/Medicaid payments. Also check the doctor's accessibility and convenience, such as office hours, waiting time to get an appointment and waiting time when you come to the office. If it is a group practice, find out whether you can see a doctor other than the one you usually see without being considered a new patient.

Your doctor should be medically qualified. Equally important, your doctor should be someone that you trust and feel comfortable talking to. Your doctor may be hindered in making a diagnosis if the 2 of you do not communicate well. If you feel unable to do this with your current doctor, consider switching doctors.

2 What is a primary care physician?

A primary care physician can help you with a wide range of medical problems, including routine physicals, special vaccines and immunizations. He or she can also make referrals to a specialist when specific problems arise. Primary care physicians are licensed as general practitioners, internists, family practitioners or pediatricians. Osteopaths are also fully licensed primary care physicians but they are licensed as DOs (Doctors of Osteopathy) rather than as MDs (Medical Doctors).

3 Why do I need a primary care doctor?

Establishing a rapport with a primary care physician can provide **consistency** in your medical treatment and help control costs.

A primary care doctor **tends to have lower fees** than specialists and can treat a wide range of problems. Rather than change from specialist to specialist each time a different problem arises, a visit to your primary care doctor can **pinpoint the problem.** Primary care physicians may also be more aware of how a new problem relates to previous conditions you have had, enabling him or her to treat it appropriately. They are in charge of seeing the **whole system.** If special consultation is needed, your primary care physician will make a referral to a specialist.

While a specialist can provide necessary consultations, your primary care physician may be able to **oversee the actual treatment.** This should reduce the necessity of follow-up visits to the specialist, whose fees may be higher than your primary care physician. Your primary care physician can always contact the specialist by phone for further advice.

You **can save money on tests and x-rays.** Your primary care physician will have your complete medical history that will contain the results of previous tests and x-rays. These records can be easily forwarded to a specialist if necessary and will avoid duplication of tests and reduce your cost.

One of the most important functions of a primary care physician is to **help reduce your anxiety** about health care and the medical field. Many primary care physicians stress preventive medicine and are trained in psychology or counseling. In addition, they can offer: **advice and reassurance** over the telephone; squeeze you in for **emergency appointments; assistance with** your health insurance; assistance in **controlling health care costs** by making sure that you do not stay in the hospital longer than necessary or providing alternatives to a hospital stay such as outpatient surgery.

4 What are the different types of primary care physicians?

All primary care physicians are trained to deal with a wide range of problems. The main distinction among them is the emphasis of their specialized training, completed during their residency.

General Internists are trained to take care of the medical problems of adults, generally treatments that do not involve surgery. Internal medicine is the study of the various organs and body systems, such as infectious diseases. Many doctors limit their practice to one of these systems, so it may be difficult to find a *true* general internist. However, many trained in a specialty also practice general medicine.

Primary Care Internists have specialized training that emphasizes the treatment of the whole patient, focusing not only on the internal body systems but their interrelationships as well.

Family Practitioners have specialized training in which they learn about all age groups as well as problems that might be caused by family dynamics. Family practitioners can provide routine care for infants as well as adults. Some family practitioners have admitting privileges at hospitals, while others do not. If you are considering a family practitioner as your primary care physician, check if he or she has hospital privileges. If not, the family practitioner will have to refer you to an internist or specialist when you require hospitalization.

Pediatricians treat the medical problems of children, from infancy to around the age of 18. Many have psychological training to treat child development and behavior problems along with physical ailments. For example, if a child complains of frequent stomachaches every morning before going to school, the pediatrician is aware that this may be a physical problem closely tied to an emotional one. Some pediatricians also specialize in adolescent medicine, which focuses on problems unique to adolescence.

Doctors of Osteopathy (DOs), also referred to as **Osteopathic physicians,** have similar training to an MD, including 4 years of college, 4 years of osteopathic medicine and then a hospital based residency. Their philosophic attitude about illness and disease differs from MDs. They are trained to do **OMT, osteopathic manipulative therapy,** which involves manipulations of the spine and is used as a diagnostic procedure and as treatment. DOs can specialize in the same fields as MDs, such as OB/GYN or radiology, and 86 percent provide primary care. In addition, they emphasize preventive medicine, proper diet and fitness.

Chiropractors base their practice on the belief that most medical problems stem from abnormalities of the spine, and treatment is based on manipulations of the spine. Chiropractors attend a 4-year chiropractic school. State laws vary on the restrictions of a chiropractor's practice. Some states limit a chiropractor to dealing only with manipulation of the spine for relief of musculoskeletal problems, while others permit a full range of primary care.

5 *What are the special considerations for women?*

Until fairly recently, many women have divided their medical care between a primary care physician and a gynecologist. However, women patients and medical professionals are reconsidering this division of women's health care. In choosing a primary physician, women should also ask, *Do you do routine gynecology?*

If you see a gynecologist for primary care, be sure that he or she does a breast examination and checks your blood pressure.

For further information on women's health care, **The New Our Bodies, Our Selves,** The Boston Women's Health Collective, Simon & Schuster, 1230 Avenue of the Americas, New York, NY 10020 and **Womancare,** Madgras & Patterson, Avon, 959 Eighth Avenue, New York, NY 10022.

6 *What are the different types of specialists?*

Allergist treats asthma, hay fever, eczema, certain skin disorders; some specialize in only one allergy.

Cardiologist specializes in heart diseases and disorders; some internists are also cardiologists and vice versa.

Dermatologist specializes in diseases of the skin.

Endocrinologist specializes in metabolic disturbances, especially diabetes and obesity.

Gastroenterologist specializes in the GI (gastro-intestinal) tract (stomach and intestines).

Gynecologist treats the female reproductive system. Some, but not all, offer obstetric care, in which case they are called **OB/GYN (obstetrician/gynecologist).**

Hematologist specializes in blood disorders.

Internist involves cardiovascular disease, endocrinology and metabolism, gastroenterology, hematology, hypertension, infectious disease, medical oncology, nephrology, pulmonary disease and rheumatology. Most specialize in one of these areas.

Nephrologist specializes in diseases of the kidney.

Neurologist specializes in diseases of the nervous system and brain disorders.

Obstetrician provides prenatal care and delivers babies. See **Gynecologist.**

Oncologist specializes in cancer. Most specialize in a particular type.

Otorhinolaryngologist specializes in ears, nose and throat. Often referred to as the **ENT** doctor.

Pathologist specializes in the study of diseases.

Pediatrician treats infants and children, usually until the age of 18.

Plastic Surgeon does cosmetic and reconstructive surgery, such as skin grafts, *nose jobs,* breast augmentations.

Proctologist specializes in colon and rectal disorders.

Pulmonary Specialist specializes in diseases of the lungs.

Radiologist specializes in reading x-rays and treatments involving radiation.

Rheumatologist specializes in arthritis.

Urologist specializes in problems of the urinary tract and kidneys. Some specialize in diseases of the prostate.

Cost of Decision

In making medical decisions today, do you take the cost of treatment into account more, about the same, or less than you did five years ago?

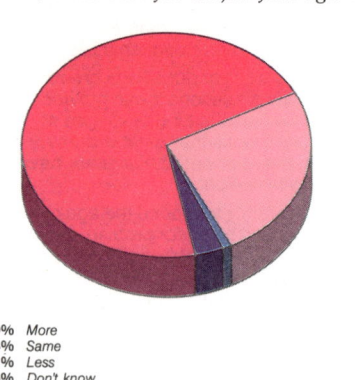

- **69%** More
- **24%** Same
- **1%** Less
- **6%** Don't know

Patient Visits *per physician per week*

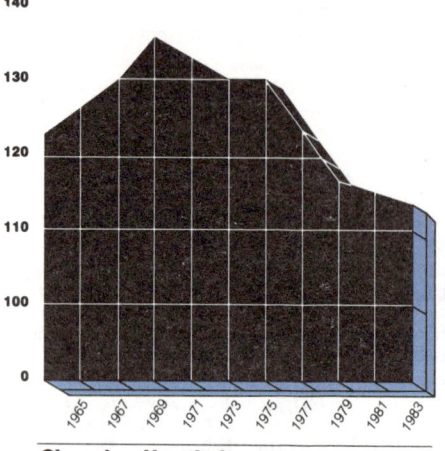

Women in Medical Schools *% of graduates*

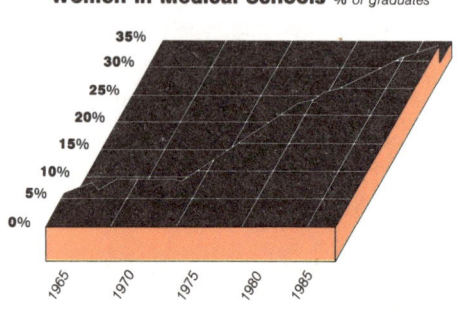

Source: American Association of Medical Colleges, August 1984

Choosing Hospitals *who decides?*

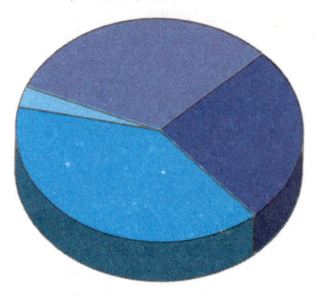

- **35%** Patients decision
- **34%** Joint decision/ doctor & patient
- **23%** Doctors decision
- **8%** Don't know

Patient Visits *by specialty*

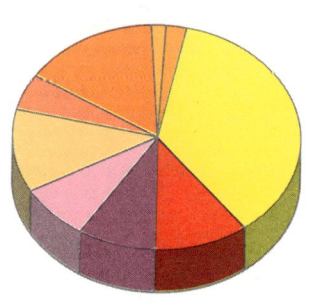

- **32.9%** General & family practice
- **16.0%** Other surgical specialties
- **12.4%** Internal Medicine
- **11.1%** Pediactrics
- **9.4%** Obstetrics & Gynecology
- **7.5%** Other medical specialties
- **5.3%** General surgery
- **2.7%** Psychiatry
- **2.7%** All other Surgical specialities

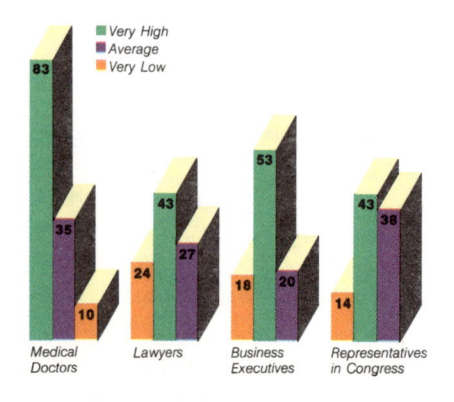

Average Expenses *self employed physicians*

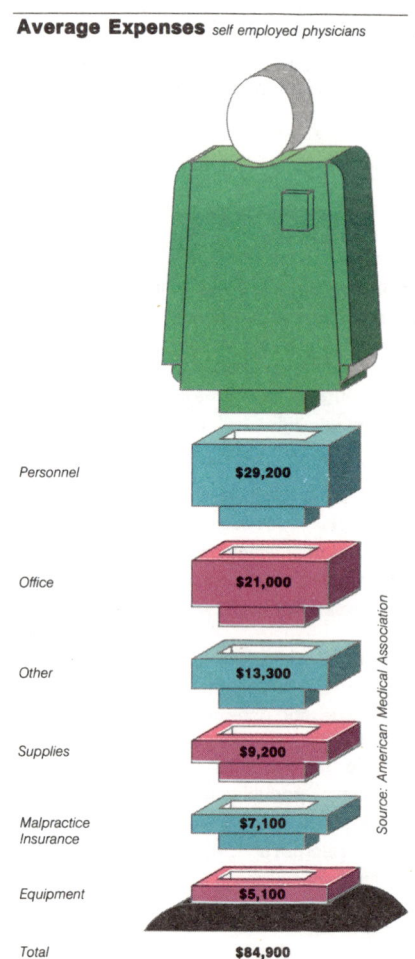

Personnel	$29,200
Office	$21,000
Other	$13,300
Supplies	$9,200
Malpractice Insurance	$7,100
Equipment	$5,100
Total	$84,900

Source: American Medical Association

Honesty & Ethical Standards *by %*

- Very High
- Average
- Very Low

Medical Doctors: 83, 35, 10
Lawyers: 24, 43, 27
Business Executives: 18, 53, 20
Representatives in Congress: 14, 43, 38

7 *What is preventive medicine?*

Preventive medicine is accepting the ultimate responsibility for our health. If we own a valuable automobile, we care for it by getting it tuned and oiled. We listen intently for buzzes and sputters; we know when it needs help. Preventive medicine encourages us to do the same with our bodies by staying fit, eating a balanced diet and diagnosing disease early. This concept represents a shift in attitude in the medical and health care fields. It is essential for all of us to educate ourselves about our health in order to intercept illness and help the medical profession serve us better.

8 *What should I know about my doctor?*

The following are ways to determine your doctor's qualifications:

Where did the doctor attend **medical school?**

Where did the doctor do his or her **residency training?**

Is the doctor **licensed** by the state licensing board and does he or she have **board certification?**

Does the doctor have **hospital staff and/or teaching appointments?** (This is more likely for a specialist.)

At which hospitals does the doctor have **admitting privileges?** This is important because it will determine where you would be hospitalized, if necessary. If a doctor has privileges at more than one hospital, then you probably would have a choice.

9 *What are 7 resources for finding a doctor and checking his or her qualifications?*

1. **Relatives, friends or co-workers** are often a good way to find a physician. Ask people whom you trust to suggest a physician or if they know anything about a doctor you are considering.

2. **Local or state medical association directories** are organized by county or large city. They will often include educational and biographical data as well as photographs. For example, in Los Angeles, the LA County Medical Association provides such information.

3. **Local hospitals or medical schools** will often make referrals. They can also advise you if the doctor accepts Medicare/Medicaid, speaks a foreign language or has a group practice.

4. **Directory of Medical Specialists,** A. N. Marquis Company, 200 E. Ohio Street, Chicago, IL 60611, 312-787-2008, is a comprehensive listing of physicians certified by the 23 specialty boards of the American Board of Specialists, published by *Who's Who.*

5. **The American Medical Directory,** American Medical Association, 535 N. Dearborn Street, Chicago, IL 60610, 312-751-6000, provides biographical information from the AMA Physicians Masterfile and contains both current and historical information on approximately 500,000 physicians, whether or not they are AMA members. Also check your library for availability.

6. **State medical quality assurance boards** can tell you if your doctor has been brought up on any charges and the nature of those charges. Find out if the doctor was actually found guilty. There has been a tremendous increase in the number of suits filed against doctors that may reflect changes in attitudes of lawyers and patients rather than a decrease in quality in the medical profession.

7. **Interview and talk to the doctor.** The small charge, if any, is worth assuring your comfort and trust.

In 1983, 16 malpractice claims were filed for every 100 doctors. (AMA internal report, quoted in NY Times, 17 Jan 1985.)

WHAT TO DO IF SURGERY HAS BEEN RECOMMENDED

10 *How urgent is the surgery?*

Surgeries fall into 2 main categories: **elective** and **emergency** (non-elective). Elective surgery is an operation or surgical procedure for a condition that is not considered to be an emergency or life threatening. Patients can sometimes choose whether or not to have this type of surgery.

11 *What 4 things should I do next?*

1. Determine what, if any, **non-surgical treatments are available.**
2. Determine the **consequences of postponing** the surgery.
3. Get a **second opinion.**
4. Also consider the **costs** and **risks versus the benefits** for any treatment, including surgery.

Costs & Risks

Possibility of infection associated with diagnostic tests or surgical procedure.

Side effects from therapies such as drug or radiation.

Loss of time from work.

Out-of-pocket payments for services not covered by your insurance policy.

Benefits

Prolonging your life.

Relief of painful symptoms.

Increasing your functional capacity. For example, if you have limited range of motion in your knee due to an injury, will the surgery enable you to participate in more activities?

12 Why should I get a second opinion?

Surgery or **hospitalization may not be necessary,** and the surgery may **result in other complications.** If surgery is necessary, another opinion will **verify** and/or give you more confidence about **your first physician's opinion.** The second physician may also shed more light on the situation.

Other forms of treatment may be appropriate. For example, a chronic knee problem may be treated with physical therapy before performing an operation, or scoliosis (curvature of the spine) can often be treated with brace therapy before a radical surgical procedure is performed.

According to the **Cornell-New York Hospital second opinion elective surgery program***, one-third of all hysterectomies and two-thirds of all tonsillectomies performed are unnecessary. Surgery for orthopedic, urologic and gynecological conditions are most frequently determined unnecessary.*

Twenty-seven percent of the patients screened at **Blue Cross/Blue Shield of Greater New York Program for Elective Surgical Second Opinion (PRESSO)** *were not confirmed for surgery. In other words, a second doctor told these patients that they did not need to have the recommended operation.*

13 What are 7 ways to get a second opinion?

Although you may feel uncomfortable, it is important to get a second opinion. Your insurance may make it mandatory.

1. **Ask your doctor** for the name of another physician, or you may prefer to find someone with no connection to your original doctor.
2. **Contact your local hospital or medical school** for the name of a specialist on staff.
3. **Ask relatives, friends, neighbors or coworkers** for suggestions or to describe their past experiences.
4. **Contact the local medical society or an appropriate health agency,** such as the American Cancer Society or American Diabetes Association.
5. **Call the Second Surgical Opinion Hot-line,** sponsored by the US government, 800-638-6833, 800-492-6603 (in Maryland).
6. **Call Cornell-New York Hospital second opinion elective surgery,** 800-522-0036, 800-631-1220 (in New York).
7. **Write for** a free booklet: **Facing Surgery? Why Not Get a Second Opinion?** Surgery Health and Human Services, 3rd & Independence SW, Washington DC 20201.

14 Do the savings of obtaining a second opinion outweigh the costs?

According to the **Cornell-New York Second Opinion Panel for Elective Surgery,** for every $1.00 spent to obtain a second opinion consultation, $2.63 was **saved** in **deferred hospital costs** and **surgeon bills, lost work days** and **other surgery-related costs.** Many insurance companies will pay for the cost of the second opinion consultation.

15 What if the second opinion conflicts with the first?

The decision to have surgery is up to you. If the second physician does not recommend surgery or recommends an alternative treatment, patients tend to follow the advice of the second physician. **Cornell-New York Hospital second opinion elective surgery program** has found that **75 percent of the patients who are not recommended for surgery never have surgery.**

Some insurance companies require that both physicians confirm the need for certain surgeries before reimbursing you. Other companies require a second opinion but leave the final decision to you if the 2 physicians do not agree.

You may want to arrange for the 2 doctors to confer so that you understand their different perspectives. Or, you may want to get a third opinion though your insurance company may not cover the consultation.

16 What 10 questions should I ask?

1. What are the **risks of performing** this procedure?
2. What are the **risks of delaying** the procedure?
3. Can it be **performed** on an **outpatient basis?**
4. Does my **primary care physician perform** the actual procedure **or a specialist?**
5. How often does the surgeon perform this surgery? (There is **less risk** with a **surgeon who has performed this surgery several times** before and who **performs it on a regular basis.**)
6. What is the **recovery time?**
7. **How soon** will I be able to walk, drive and **return to my daily routine?**
8. What are the **post-operative procedures,** such as follow-up treatment, physical therapy or special exercises?
9. Will I need **special help at home?**
10. What are the **estimated costs** of the surgery and hospital stay?

17 What is outpatient surgery?

When a procedure is performed on an **outpatient** basis, the patient enters the hospital or an ambulatory care facility in the morning. The procedure is performed, and the patient is generally discharged later the same day. Surgeries performed on an outpatient basis are less complex than major procedures that require prolonged post-operative monitoring and hospital care to

18 What are 3 types of outpatient facilities?

An **ambulatory care facility** is equipped to deal with all the necessary pre-operative, operative and post-operative procedures that do not require an overnight stay in the hospital.

There are 2 types of **hospital-based** programs. Both are within the hospital structure. If any complications develop, there is no need for a transfer. In the first one, called **hospital based-nondedicated unit,** the patient is admitted to the hospital, the surgery is performed, and the patient is discharged directly from the recovery room when his or her condition warrants it. The patient never occupies a bed in the hospital. The second type, **hospital based-defined unit,** is similar to inpatient surgery because the patient must go through the same administrative procedures and occupies a regular bed after the procedure. The patient is released without an overnight stay, unless complications develop. This cuts some costs but may be more expensive than a nondedicated unit or a freestanding facility.

A **freestanding unit or surgi-center** is separate from other health care facilities and may be administered by a group of surgeons, by a hospital or even a group of businesspeople in consultation with surgeons. It provides **convenient, one-stop patient care**, from admission to pre-operative procedures to post-operative care. A freestanding facility may be more attractive and less frightening to patients, as well as more attractive and convenient for physicians. Fees tend to be lower than hospital based units; however, the 2 types compete for clients. The disadvantage is that a freestanding facility does not have the wide range of equipment and support systems that a hospital-based unit has. If complications occur, a transfer to a nearby hospital is required. Also, you must be examined by a physician before leaving a freestanding facility.

19 What types of procedures can be performed?

A wide variety of procedures can be performed on an outpatient basis, such as: **removal of cysts; biopsy; repair of facial wounds; dilation and curettage (D & C); orthopedic procedures,** such as application of a cast or exploratory surgery (such as an arthroscopy); **surgery for varicose saphenous veins; blepharoplasty** (eyelid surgery).

If you have a recently written insurance policy, some of these procedures will only be covered by your insurance if they are performed on an outpatient basis. Check if there is coverage for procedures performed on an outpatient basis.

20 What are 4 advantages?

1. It is **less expensive** because you do not spend the night in the hospital, and as mentioned, some insurance companies will only cover the procedure if it is performed on an outpatient basis.

2. It helps to **prevent family disruptions**.

3. It **reduces the psychological trauma** of having an operation.

4. Often, there is **earlier recovery** in familiar surroundings.

21 What are 5 other considerations?

1. Make sure your **general health is good enough not to need** the resources of a hospital if you are having the surgery performed at an ambulatory care center or clinic.

2. Determine if there is an **advantage to being in the hospital** in case you need to stay overnight.

3. Make arrangements for **assistance to get home.** You may be groggy from a general anesthetic or limited in mobility by bandages or a cast.

4. Be sure the **facility is accredited** by the **Accreditation Association for Ambulatory Health Care**, 9933 Lawler Avenue, Skokie, IL 60077, 312-676-9610.

5. If the procedure is performed at a freestanding facility, find out **what arrangements it has for transfer to a hospital** if it becomes necessary.

22 Can I refuse treatment?

Yes. **You can refuse hospitalization or treatment**, but you must be fully aware of the consequences of your refusal. Ask your doctor what the implications of refusing a particular treatment will be. Find out if your refusal is life-threatening, if it will lead to a slow degradation or worsening of a problem, or if it is only a temporary inconvenience. Also check that your insurance company will pay subsequent bills if you refuse a treatment or procedure. Then make your decision.

HOSPITALS

You will usually go to the hospital where your doctor is on staff. If your doctor is on staff at more than one hospital, you have a choice. If you do not like the hospital(s) where your doctor is on staff, you may have to decide between the hospital you prefer and the doctor you prefer. It is good to know ahead of time about the different kinds of hospitals and which one is best for a particular ailment. Hospitals vary in size and quality. For each type of hospital, you will want to know: the patient/staff ratio, visiting hours, the type of staff on duty at night and any other special requirements that are important to you. For example, if you want your husband to be with you during the delivery of your baby, check if the hospital allows this. You can obtain this information from the admitting office.

23 What are the different types of hospitals?

Teaching hospitals are often affiliated with a university and concern themselves with teaching and research. If you have a difficult or unusual illness, this might be the best place because it will often have specialists on hand, the latest technology and students (interns or residents) who may be able to take a special interest in your case. You can refuse to participate in an experimental program at a teaching hospital. The main disadvantage to a teaching hospital is the lack of privacy.

Private hospitals are run for profit and may be owned by a private group, religious group or corporation. Groups such as **American Medical International (AMI), Hospital Corporation of America (HCA)** and **Humana** which own multi-hospital systems, have grown immensely over the past several years. This may enable them to provide services at a lower cost due to **economy of scale.** Investor-owned corporations can own teaching hospitals also. Ask friends and relatives about a hospital's reputation.

Community hospitals are usually non-profit, tax-supported facilites. They may offer less specialization than the teaching hospital, though they may be better suited for more routine care.

Special care hospitals specialize in treating specific diseases or types of patients, such as cancer, psychiatric, cardiology or women and children.

There are also **government and veteran's administration (VA) hospitals** that provide care for veterans.

Some facilities specialize in **long term convalescent** care. **Hospices,** for example, specialize in the care of terminally ill patients, incorporating the philosophy that supportive health care should be given to make a patient's last days more pleasant. Hospice care may be based in a facility or geared to the patient's home, depending on the patient's condition.

24 What are 7 reasons for hospitalization?

1. **Diagnostic test**
2. **Observation**
3. **Surgery**
4. **Delivery of a baby**
5. **Quarantine for communicable disease**
6. **Mental Health**
7. **Detoxification or problems related to substance abuse.**

IN THE HOSPITAL

25 What arrangements should I make?

If you are going in for **elective surgery,** determine the most convenient time for your hospitalization and recovery period. Hospitals may be short staffed during weekends and major holidays such as Christmas and New Years. Check when the hospital has a new group of residents and interns (usually in July); you may want to wait until they have worked themselves into the hospital routine.

Ask your physician or call the admitting office to **determine which lab tests can be done on an outpatient basis** beforehand. You should also discuss with the admitting office your preference for a room, whether **VIP, private, semi-private, ward or smoking/nonsmoking.** A VIP suite usually has a seating area, desk and more decorative interior. Find out what day and at what time you are scheduled for admission.

Take any precautionary measures to protect your home as if you were going out of town.

26 Should I get a private room?

Private rooms are more expensive, and often your **insurance policy only covers semi-private rooms;** you will have to pay the difference. But, if you cherish your privacy, then the extra expense is probably worthwhile. A **semi-private** or **ward situation may be advantageous** for the very sick or eldery, patients with poor vision or hearing impairment and patients without family or a companion, because they can benefit from a roommate's watchful eye. Even short hospital stays can be lonely.

For **children,** private rooms offer parents a chance to room-in, while wards give children with long hospital stays playmates and companions. Some hospitals have special sleeping accommodations for parents as well as special play areas for children.

27 How can I prepare my child?

The hospital can be a large, unfamiliar place, especially for children. The more you tell children, the more you can relieve their fears and anxieties in order to gain and maintain their trust.

Some hospitals have **pre-admission tours or programs** for you and your child. If your hospital does not have such a program, see what you can find out for your child ahead of time. The information that a child needs to know is not very different from the kind of information that an adult would like to know.

Children have special medical needs. Check a hospital's **pediatric department** in the same way that you might check a coronary care unit for a patient with heart disease. There are also hospitals that specialize only in children and children's diseases.

By explaining the following 5 areas, you can allay your child's fears and anxieties.

1. **Describe** what the **tests** will be like.
2. **Describe** what the **surgery** will be like.
3. **Describe** the **hospital room** if you are unable to go there before your child is admitted.
4. **Describe** what the **equipment** does.
5. **Explain** who the different **staff members** are and what they do.

Encourage your child to ask questions and answer them honestly. If you do not know the answer, ask your child's doctor.

Shots Children Should Have
The American Academy of Pediatrics has set these guidelines for children's vaccinations:

Age	Vaccine	Method	Age	Vaccine	Method	Age	Vaccine	Method
2 mos	Diptheria	Injection	4 mos	Diptheria	Injection	1.5 yrs	Diptheria	Injection
	Tetanus	Injection		Tetanus	Injection		Tetanus	Injection
	Whooping			Whooping			Whooping	
	Cough	Injection		Cough	Injection		Cough	Injection
	Polio	Oral		Polio	Oral		Polio	Oral
			6 mos	Diptheria	Injection	4-6	Diptheria	Injection
				Tetanus	Injection		Tetanus	Injection
				Whooping			Whooping	
				Cough	Injection		Cough	Injection
							Polio	Injection
			15 mos	Measles	Injection	14-16	Diptheria	Injection
				Mumps	Injection		Tetanus	Injection
				Rubella	Injection			

28 *What should I bring to the hospital?*

Many patients feel more comfortable in the hospital if they bring a few reminders from home with them such as:

1. a **photograph** of family members
2. an inexpensive **vase** (the hospital is usually in short supply)
3. loose fitting, **comfortable clothing**
4. a **cassette player** with earphones
5. if you prefer **your own pillow,** make sure you have a distinct pillowcase to identify it
6. **reading material** such as books or magazines
7. **games**

You should also bring little **necessities from home** to avoid buying them from the hospital:

8. **toothbrush and toothpaste**
9. **brush and comb**
10. **shaving cream, razors and aftershave**
11. **perfume and make-up**
12. **robe** and **slippers** with skid-proof soles

Also bring:

13. your medical **insurance card and information**
14. your **Social Security number**
15. **medical records and histories** if you have them
16. **names, telephone numbers and addresses of family and friends** who may need to be contacted

Don't bring valuables. Leave your jewelry at home and carry only a few dollars in cash.

29 *What forms will I be asked to sign?*

Unless you are an emergency patient, you will go directly to the admitting office to fill out several different forms that are designed to protect you, the physician and the hospital. **Know what you are signing and why.**

You are legally entitled to **informed consent.** Your physician is responsible for providing you with a **thorough and understandable description** of what is going to happen to you. However, your doctor's concept of what is understandable may differ from your perception. **Ask questions** to make sure you understand everything. Your physician is the best person to describe the procedures to be performed and the risks involved. **Knowing the risks** is an important part of being properly informed. **DON'T BE INTIMIDATED!**

30 *What is informed consent?*

To be **legally informed,** your doctor should have spent enough time with you to make you feel that:

1. You **understand your medical condition.**
2. You **understand the basic procedure** to be performed.
3. You are **aware of any alternative treatment** available, whether surgical or non-surgical.
4. You **understand the benefits and the risks** involved with the recommended procedures, including those **risks involved with anesthesia.**
5. You can **reject the treatment** suggested with knowledge of the risks.

31 *Do I have to sign these forms?*

The first form you will most likely be presented with is a **standard form** upon entering the hospital. **You must sign to be admitted.** The California form is typical and covers these factors:

1. You are **responsible for your hospital bill.**
2. You must **authorize your insurance company to pay** your hospital bill.
3. The hospital accepts **only certain health care plans.**
4. The hospital may **release information to whoever is paying your bill.**
5. The hospital is **not responsible for your valuables** unless placed in the hospital safe.
6. You must **arrange for any special nursing** requirements. The hospital gives you only general nursing care.

Any surgery will require a **consent form** that authorizes a certain surgeon to perform a specific surgery. Read the form carefully, and make sure you understand all about the surgery before signing.

You may encounter other forms, depending on your treatment.

32 What is an Intensive Care Unit (ICU)?

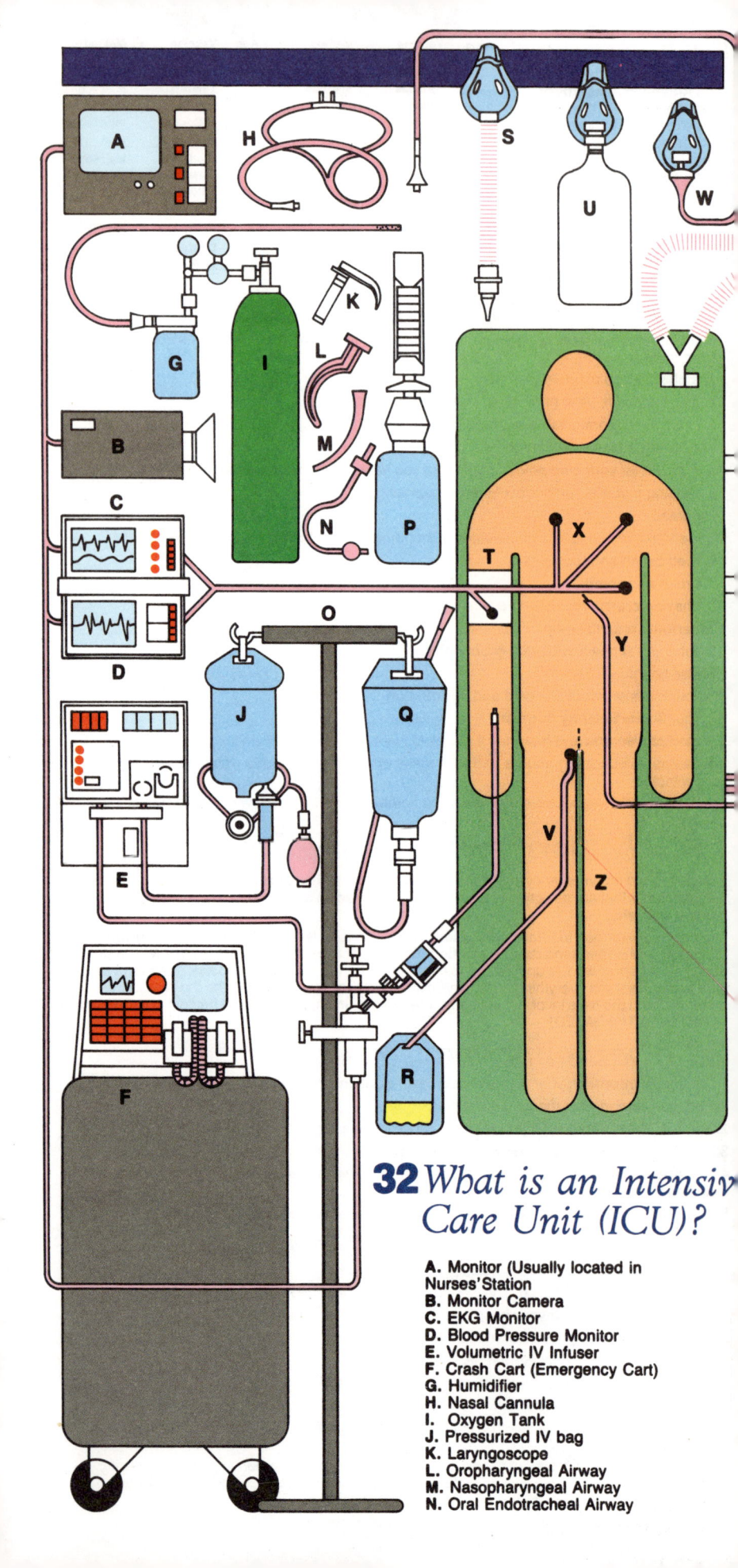

A. Monitor (Usually located in Nurses' Station
B. Monitor Camera
C. EKG Monitor
D. Blood Pressure Monitor
E. Volumetric IV Infuser
F. Crash Cart (Emergency Cart)
G. Humidifier
H. Nasal Cannula
I. Oxygen Tank
J. Pressurized IV bag
K. Laryngoscope
L. Oropharyngeal Airway
M. Nasopharyngeal Airway
N. Oral Endotracheal Airway

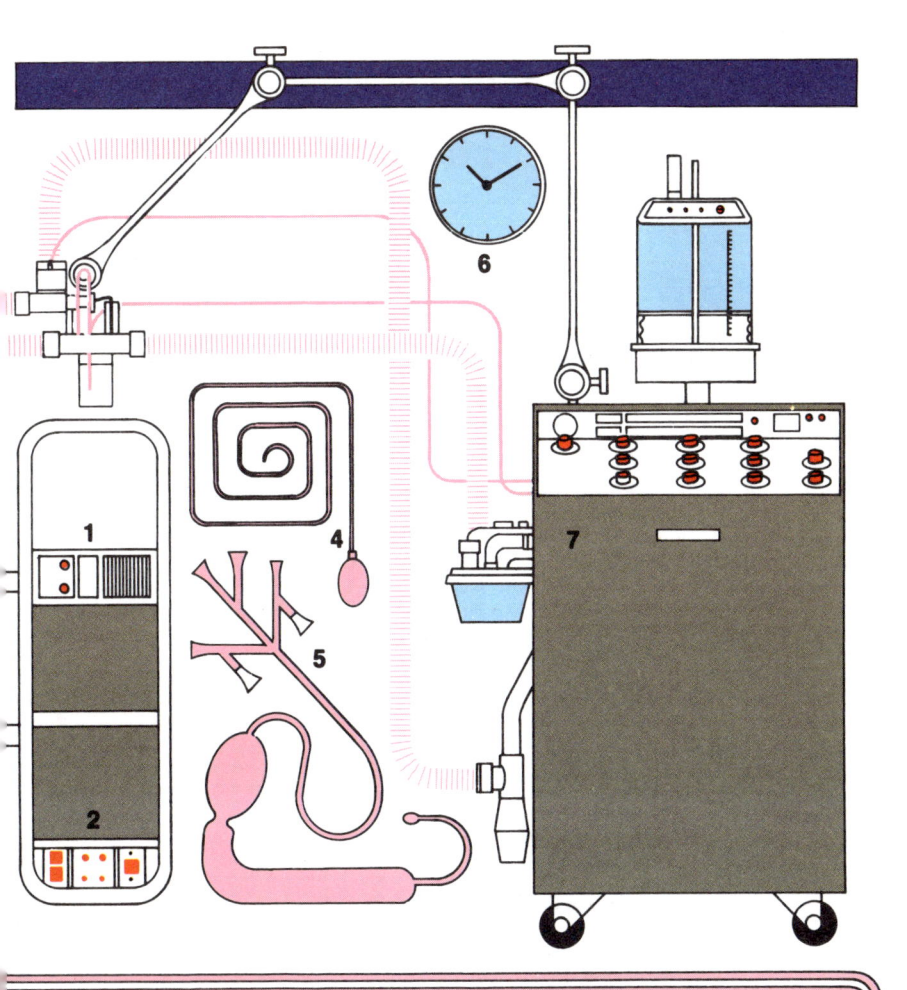

O. IV Stand
P. Wall-Mounted Oxygen Source
Q. Enteric Feeding Bag
R. Foley Urine Collection Bag
S. Venturi Mask
T. Blood Pressure Cuff
U. Partial Rebreathing Mask
V. Urinary Catheter
W. Low-Flow Mask
X. EKG Leads
Y. Thoracic Drainage
Z. Rectal Temperature Monitor

1. Bedside Telephone
2. Bed Controls; Nurses' Call Button
3. Thoracic Drainage Unit
4. Cantor Intestinal Tube
5. Esophagogastric Tamponade Tube
6. Real Time Clock
7. Ventilator (Respiratory Assistance and Treatment)
8. Hypo-Hyper Thermia Core Temperature Regulator

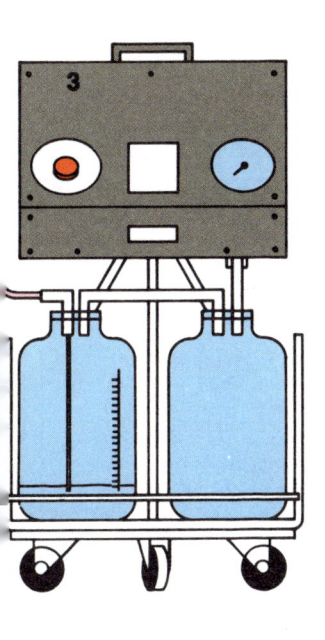

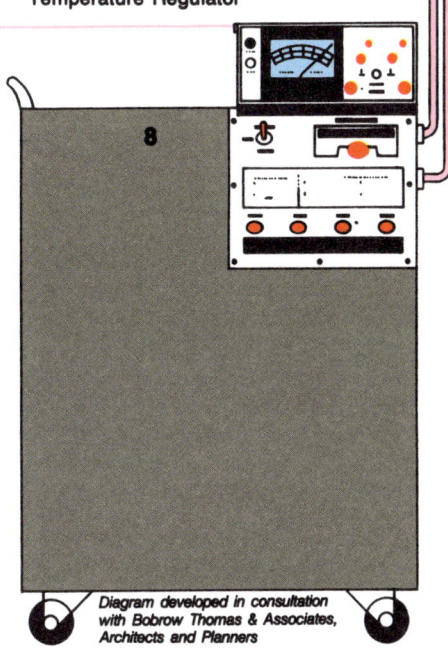

Diagram developed in consultation with Bobrow Thomas & Associates, Architects and Planners

33 What is an Operating Room (OR)?

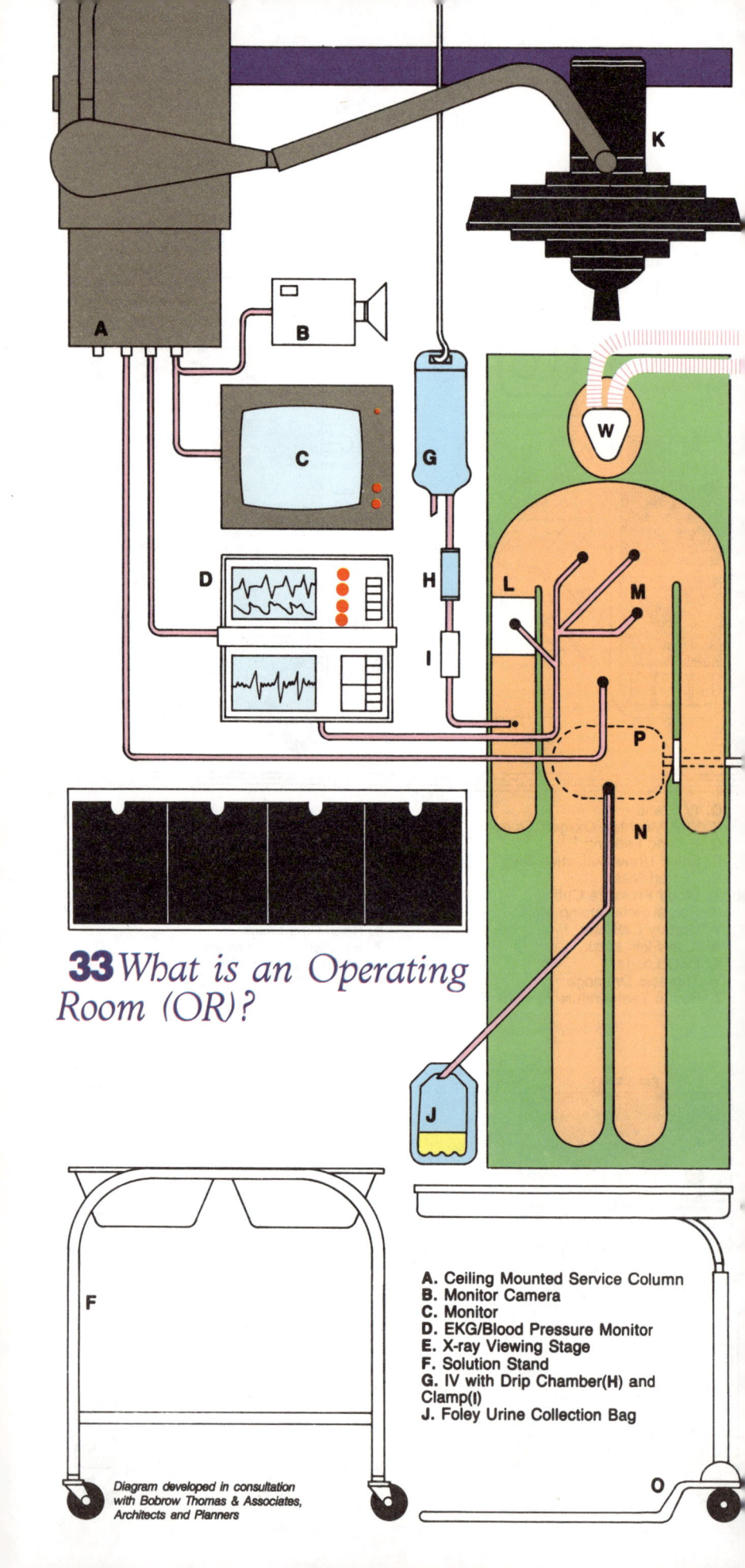

A. Ceiling Mounted Service Column
B. Monitor Camera
C. Monitor
D. EKG/Blood Pressure Monitor
E. X-ray Viewing Stage
F. Solution Stand
G. IV with Drip Chamber(**H**) and Clamp(**I**)
J. Foley Urine Collection Bag

Diagram developed in consultation with Bobrow Thomas & Associates, Architects and Planners

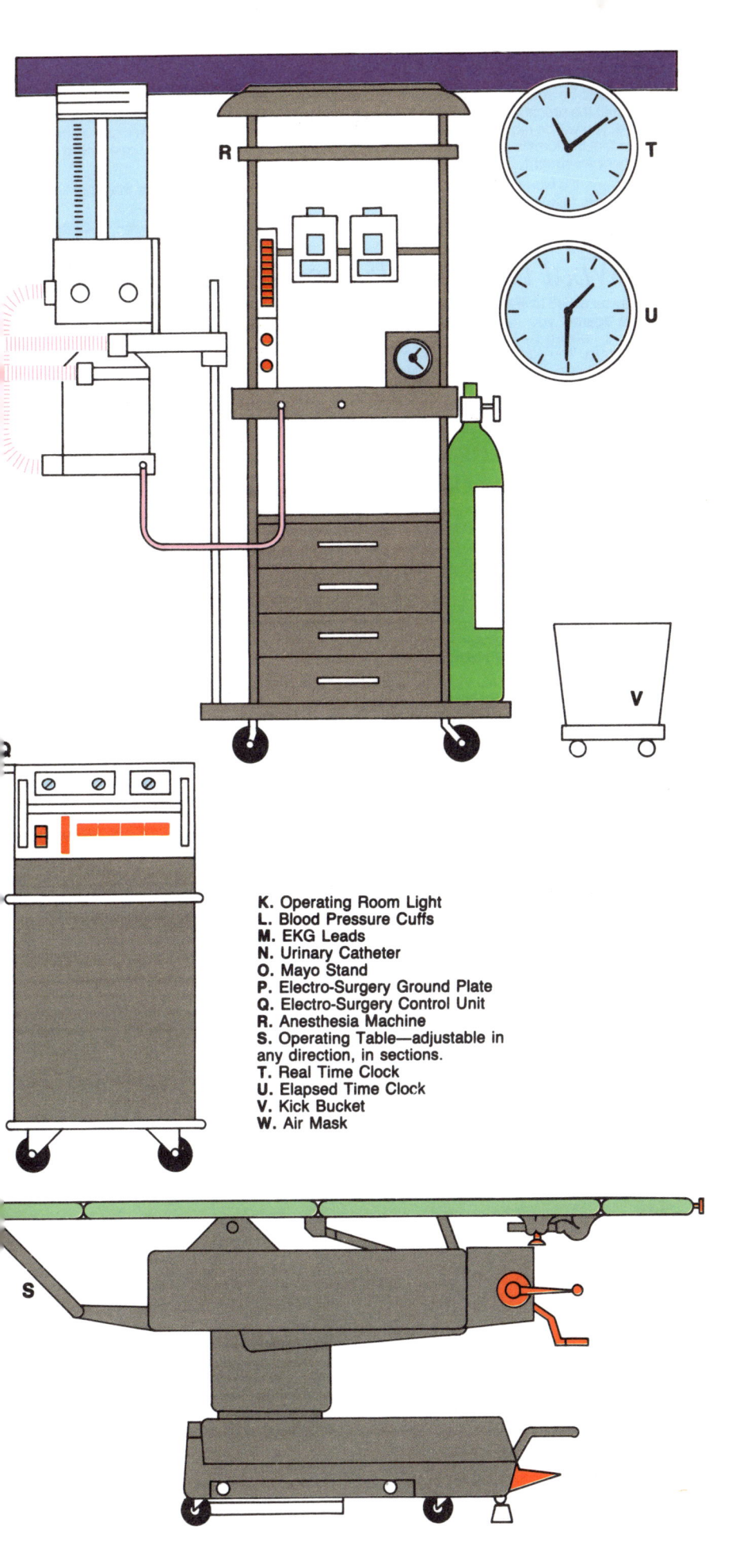

K. Operating Room Light
L. Blood Pressure Cuffs
M. EKG Leads
N. Urinary Catheter
O. Mayo Stand
P. Electro-Surgery Ground Plate
Q. Electro-Surgery Control Unit
R. Anesthesia Machine
S. Operating Table—adjustable in any direction, in sections.
T. Real Time Clock
U. Elapsed Time Clock
V. Kick Bucket
W. Air Mask

34 What if I am having a diagnostic test?

If you need to be admitted to the hospital for a **diagnostic test**, it is probably an **invasive test** which means that the procedure **introduces tubes or probes into your body**. Because there is some risk involved, you will be required to sign a **consent form**. Again, know what you are signing and why. Be sure that the form is **only for the diagnostic procedure so that decisions concerning further surgery or treatment, if necessary, can be discussed with you**.

For example, if a woman has a breast biopsy and the doctor finds a larger tumor than expected, he or she should perform the biopsy only, not a radical mastectomy.

If you change your mind and no longer want to have a certain procedure performed, have the signed consent form returned to you.

35 What is an arbitration agreement?

You may be asked to sign an **arbitration agreement**. Under this system, any malpractice claim that you file against your doctor will be handled by an **arbitration panel** of 3 arbitrators, 1 chosen by you, 1 chosen by the physician and third chosen by the other 2 arbitrators, **rather than going to court**. The panel presides over a hearing which you attend with or without your lawyer, and which the physician and a representative attend. The panel then decides the verdict which is binding for you and your doctor. **You do not have to sign this form.**

Arbitration can save you court costs and **a lengthy wait for a court date** but **may result in a lower settlement**. Several states have approved arbitration for the medical field.

Make sure you fully understand the process before deciding to sign an arbitration agreement.

36 After I fill out these forms, then what?

A staff person in the admitting office will take information on your medical insurance, your personal and family medical history and other pertinent information about yourself.

It is best to make arrangements ahead of time, but if you have not, now is the time to ask about room types. If you smoke, or if you do not smoke and object to it, say so before you are assigned a roommate.

You will also receive an **identification bracelet** which has your name and the name of the attending physician on it. Never try to take it off. Generally, nurses are required to check your ID bracelet before giving you any medication. If you are having surgery, it is one of the ways that the nurses identify you in the recovery room.

You may receive a series of general tests, such as a **blood test, EKG** and **chest x-ray** and be asked to give a **urine sample**.

Once in your room, a nurse will record your **vital signs: blood pressure, pulse rate, respiration, temperature**. The nurse will take a more **detailed medical history**. Tell him or her about any **previous problems, allergies to food** or **drugs, reactions to drugs or doctor's restrictions**, particularly if the physician is not directly involved with the surgical procedure or hospital stay.

37 What is my schedule during my stay?

Hospitals start bustling early in the morning. If you do not have to be awakened early, and would like to sleep late, check with your nurse to see if this is possible. Otherwise, the hospital day goes something like this:

6:00-7:00am Nursing day shift arrives.

7:00-8:00am First surgeries of the day, and physician's rounds start. Blood samples taken, if necessary.

8:00am Breakfast.

8:00am-noon Morning baths, vital signs checked, treatments, exercises, beds changed.

Noon Lunch.

1:00-5:00pm Afternoon treatments and medications.

5:00-6:00pm Dinner.

6:00-8:00pm Evening visiting hours.

8:00-10:00pm Preparations for sleep: medications, instructions to patients if tests or surgery are to be performed the next day.

In most hospitals, you will **fill out a menu** each day for the next day's meals. You will have a choice of appetizers, main courses, side dishes such as vegetables, dessert and a beverage. Some hospitals serve better food than others, but you can usually have your advocate or companion bring in food from home or a restaurant if it does not conflict with any dietary restrictions.

38 What are 7 things the anesthesiologist needs to know about my medical history?

The **anesthesiologist** will interview you before your surgery in order to determine what type of anesthesia to use. He or she should ask you the following questions. If you feel any of these questions have been overlooked, offer the information.

1. Do you have any **allergies**?

2. Do you have any **medical problems** such as heart disease, diabetes or sickle cell anemia?

3. Are you **taking any medication**?

4. Have you had **anesthesia in the past**?

5. If so, **how recently?** Some anesthesia cannot be repeated until a specific amount of time has passed.

6. Have you ever had any **adverse reactions** to anesthesia in the past, such as high fever or vomiting?

7. Do you have a **history of severe bleeding**?

39 When do the nursing shifts change?

You can generally expect to see fresh faces at approximately **7:00am, 3:00pm and 11:00pm.** Nurses are usually *in report* (telling the oncoming shift what has transpired during the previous one) for about half an hour after these times. Try to **request assistance or pain medicine before a shift change.**

40 Who will I meet in the hospital?

You will encounter a wide variety of personnel in the hospital, each with his or her own responsibilities and titles. You need to know whom you can ask which question, who will be responsible for which aspects of your care and whom to call when you need assistance.

You will encounter **nurses** the most often throughout your day. Different nurses have different qualifications, and therefore, different responsibilities. Like any relationship, your relationship with the nurses is a 2-way street: nurses understand your need for attentive care, and you need to understand that their workload may keep them from responding to you immediately.

Some units in some hospitals use a **total patient care** approach in which a nurse has the responsibility for all of the needs of the 7 or 8 patients assigned to him or her. Others use a **team** approach in which an RN acts as team leader and oversees the functions of LPNs or LVNs and aides and performs specific tasks for a large group of patients.

You can request the care of the nurse with whom you feel the most comfortable and in most cases your request will be met.

The following is a list of the **different nurses, their qualifications** and **their general responsibilities.**

Registered Nurses (RNs) are licensed nurses who have passed their state board exams. Their education may include a 2-year degree in nursing from a community college, a 3-year hospital diploma or a 4-year BS degree in nursing. They **plan your nursing care in conjunction with your attending physician** and make decisions regarding your care within the physician's plan. When needs arise that are not covered by the physician's orders, the RN will contact your attending physician.

Licensed Practical Nurses (LPNs) or **Licensed Vocational Nurses (LVNs)** work under the RN's direction and have graduated from a 1-year practical, hands-on nursing school or program. They **take temperatures, blood pressure** and **pulse and respiration rates** and record this data on your chart. They also **give injections, apply compresses, change surgical dressings** and **administer prescribed drugs.**

Nurses Aides have had limited training. They **record your vital signs** and can **help with your personal needs** such as bathing and massages.

The **head nurse**, also referred to as **nurse coordinator** or **nurse manager,** is in charge of the floor or ward and can **handle any problem you might have with nurses or other staff members.**

The head nurse reports to the nursing supervisor or the **Director of Nursing (DON).** The DON is the **senior administrator** in nursing and may also have other departments reporting to him or her. The director can **handle your last resort problems.**

You may encounter several different **doctors** depending on the nature of your case and the type of hospital you are in.

Medical students who have been in medical school for a couple of years will be assigned to you in a teaching hospital. They are there to learn and observe.

Interns, also called **first-year, post-graduate trainees** have graduated from medical school and have earned their **MD or DO degree.** They take histories, examine patients and order tests and treatments **under the supervision of more experienced physicians.**

Residents, also called **post-graduate trainees,** have **completed medical school and their intern rotation.** They will examine you and are **authorized to administer certain treatments and procedures.** They are nearing completion of their training which can last up to 6 years as they concentrate on their specialty. One may be assigned to your case.

Your **attending physician** is in charge of your case and may be either the doctor who sent you to the hospital or a **staff resident** now in charge of your case.

Other doctors you may encounter include your **surgeon,** who specializes in surgery, and an **anesthesiologist** (See question 6).

Orderlies, aides or volunteers will bring you food, bedpans or help your nurse. With their limited training, they cannot help with your medical needs, but they can **make your hospital stay more pleasant and comfortable.**

The **dietician** may meet with you to discuss a special diet. Other specially trained people include **physical therapists, recreation therapists, occupational therapists, respiratory therapists, speech therapists, lab technicians, patient educators** and **social workers.**

41 Who do I contact with questions?

You can ask your doctor, nurse or **patient's representative.** Do not feel silly about repeating questions. It is your responsibility to **ask questions until you understand.**

42 What do I need to know about policy?

You will receive a packet of information when you are admitted to the hospital that describes **hospital policy** on everything from visiting hours to special services, such as patient education seminars. The hospital should have a set policy that covers most questions. Feel free to ask about any of your concerns.

43 When are visiting hours?

Each hospital has its own **visiting hours** which usually start around 9:00 or 10:00am and last until 8:00 or 9:00pm. **Age restrictions** vary with different hospitals and within wards of a hospital.

To respect the rights of your roommate (if you have one), try not to break the rules by allowing your guests to stay extra hours. If you have a private room, the rules may be more flexible. Visiting hours vary by ward or floor. Check with your nurse if you have any questions.

The **Intensive Care Unit (ICU)** has special rules that limit the length of the visit and the number of people permitted to visit at one time. Check with the hospital.

44 Can I see my chart?

Your **chart** is where your doctor writes your **orders, medications** and **progress reports**, along with your **medical history, notes from the lab, x-ray department, nursing notes** and **surgical notes**. If you want to see your chart, discuss this with your attending physician. Although access laws vary from state to state, you are entitled to know what is on your chart.

Legally, the chart belongs to the hospital. You have the right to **review your record** and **request a copy**. You will have to pay for the costs of copying and expect to wait a reasonable time to get one; the medical records office is often very busy.

If for some reason the hospital tries to rebuff your attempts to obtain a copy of your chart, you may have to settle for reading it at the hospital. Check with the hospital administration if you are having trouble. You should be able to **get your chart transferred for another doctor to see.** If worst comes to worst, and you cannot get access to your chart, contact your lawyer.

45 Can I change doctors in the hospital?

Yes, but **try to work out the problem with your doctor.** For example, if you feel that your doctor is not communicating well by treating your questions with curt, indifferent answers, explain how you feel. You may be able to resolve the problem by calling it to his or her attention.

However, if the problem cannot be resolved, ask the doctor if there is a colleague that he or she will recommend. If the doctor is not helpful, ask your nurse or patient's representative for assistance. You may also want to contact the hospital administration.

You can always get another doctor, although you or your companion/advocate have to make arrangements for a new one.

46 When will the doctor make rounds?

Ask your doctor when his or her visits will be so you do not sit around waiting anxiously. If you are at a teaching hospital, find out if your attending physician will be present during rounds. **Save your non-urgent questions for the doctor's visit** and be sure to **write them down. During rounds, your doctor will check your progress, review any special problems** or **alter your treatment.** For example, he or she may change the dose of a certain medication or increase the amount of exercise you do each day.

Keep a notebook in which you write notes about tests performed, comments made by the doctor or nurses and any questions or comments that you would like to discuss with your doctor. Use this list to **check your bill** or as **a record if complications occur** later.

47 Why do I need an advocate?

Whether you are in the doctor's office or in the hospital, you may not be focused enough to ask the right questions or remember the answers. A **trusted friend, relative** or **companion** can act as your **advocate.** He or she can help you make informed decisions about your health care.

Your advocate should be as assertive and as strong as possible. Try to choose someone who will stand up to authority figures for you and will help you **get information about your condition, any procedures that will be performed** and **the rate of your recovery.**

He or she can also **observe changes in your condition, ask questions** and **offer moral support.**

48 What are 6 other tasks that my advocate/companion can do?

1. Help you **keep a record** of treatments, medications, lab work and any questions you want to ask your doctor.

2. **Help with your meals** by bringing food from home or a restaurant, if it does not conflict with your prescribed diet.

3. **Help with your bathing, changing sheets and massages.**

4. Talk to your doctor or nurse on your behalf and **clarify any misunderstandings.**

5. Learn to **assist you with medications** to make sure you are receiving the right dose.

6. Learn to **assist you with special equipment, treatment, diets or other special needs.**

Some of the above tasks may **save the cost of a private duty nurse** either in the hospital or upon your return home, particularly if you are in a difficult financial situation.

RIGHTS

49 What are my rights as a patient?

Your rights as a patient stem from the desire to know as much as possible about what is going to happen to your body in order to make clear decisions about the course of your treatment. It is ultimately your responsibility to ask good questions in order to receive clear information. Ask your physician to **clarify any technical or confusing explanations.**

The **American Hospital Association (AHA)** has assembled a list of rights and entitlements for patients. Your hospital may or may not abide by these suggestions; check with the admitting office. The hospital may either give you a copy of the rights in your admission packet or post it in your room. It incorporates several items which are your legal right and several others which are considered courtesies.

1. **The patient has the right to considerate and respectful care.**

Speak up if the staff calls you by a name that you dislike, or treats you in a way that seems demeaning. Many hospitals have a patient's representative to handle such complaints. Check to see if your hospital has one. If not, find out who plays this role.

2. The patient has the right to obtain from his or her physician complete current information concerning his or her diagnosis, treatment and prognosis in terms the patient can reasonably be expected to understand. When it is not medically advisable to give such information to the patient, the information should be made available to an appropriate person in his or her behalf. He or she has the right to know by name the physician responsible for coordinating his or her care.

You must be made fully aware of the consequences of your treatment. Your doctor may have difficulty explaining technical terms in understandable lay terms. It is your responsibility to ask so that you can make an informed consent. The right to know the doctor's name and to know who is responsible for your treatment is also incorporated in this statement.

3. The patient has the right to receive from his or her physician information necessary to give informed consent prior to the start of any procedure and/or treatment. Except in emergencies, such information for informed consent should include but not necessarily be limited to the specific procedure and/or treatment, the medically significant risks involved and the probable duration of incapacitation. Where medically significant alternatives for care or treatment exist, or when the patient requests information concerning medical alternatives, the patient has the right to such information. The patient also has the right to know the name of the person responsible for the procedures and/or treatment.

This further explains right #2. You clearly must know the alternatives before entering into any procedure. Ask about the alternatives, their risks and the risks of delaying the recommended procedure or treatment. This legal right to have information before agreeing to your medical procedure is based on the legal principles of contract.

4. The patient has the right to refuse treatment to the extent permitted by law and to be informed of the medical consequences of his or her action.

You have the legal right to refuse treatment that you do not think is necessary or feel is not worth the pain, trauma or expense. You are entitled to an explanation of what will happen to you if you refuse treatment. You may have to sign a release form that releases the hospital from liability. Make sure you get any signed consent forms back if you change your mind.

5. The patient has the right to every consideration of his or her privacy concerning his or her own medical care program. Case discussion, consultation, examination and treatment are confidential and should be conducted discreetly. Those not directly involved in his or her care must have the permission of the patient to be present.

This extension of the right to courteous treatment has its legal basis in the right to privacy. If you are in a teaching hospital, students will be present at your examinations. You may refuse to be examined by so many people and may refuse to be examined twice if it is not necessary.

6. The patient has the right to expect that all communication and records pertaining to his or her care should be treated as confidential.

Confidentiality is a legal requirement of the doctor/patient relationship. This may present a problem in a teaching hospital where so many people know about the details of your medical care. If you are bothered by any lack of confidentiality, talk to your doctor, then to your patient representative.

7. The patient has the right to expect that within its capacity the hospital must make reasonable response to the request of a patient for services. The hospital must provide evaluation, service and/or referral as indicated by the urgency of the case. When medically permissable, a patient may be transferred to another facility only after he or she has received complete information and explanation concerning the needs for and alternatives to such a transfer. The institution to which the patient is to be transferred must first have accepted the patient for transfer.

You should not be arbitrarily transferred at any time. If you are transferred, it should be for a good reason and not present any risk to your condition. If you are unable to pay your bill, you may be transferred to a tax-supported community hospital, particularly if you were originally admitted in an emergency situation.

8. The patient has the right to obtain information as to any relationship of his or her hospital to other health care and educational institutions insofar as his or her care is concerned. The patient has the right to obtain information as to the existence of any professional relationship among individuals, by name who are treating him or her.

Again, you should know who is treating you. A physician must have admitting privileges at a hospital in order to practice there. However, you are entitled to outside consultants if you would like them. You or your advocate have to ask for them.

9. The patient has the right to be advised if the hospital proposes to engage in or perform human experimentation affecting his or her care or treatment. The patient has the right to refuse to participate in such research projects.

It is your legal right, established in 1966, to refuse such treatment. Be as aware as possible of what your treatment involves (an advocate can help here) in order to protect yourself from experimental treatments that you do not know about. You should fully understand the risks of any experimental procedure and the alternatives.

10. The patient has the right to expect reasonable continuity of care. He or she has the right to know in advance what appointment times and physicians are available and where. The patient has the right to expect that the hospital will provide a mechanism whereby he or she is informed by his or her physician or a delegate of the physician of the patient's continuing health care requirements following discharge.

This is another extension of courtesy. The hospital should inform you of the need to make follow up appointments, whether at the hospital, clinic or at your doctor's office. Make sure you have the appropriate medication needed for your recovery, as well as a thorough explanation of how you should care for yourself. If you are going home, the hospital's discharge planner or your doctor should inform you of any special needs and help you arrange for home nursing services available through the hospital or other resources.

If you are going to a special care facility, such as a hospice or nursing home, the Social Service Department of the hospital should make those arrangements for you.

11. The patient has the right to examine and receive an explanation of his or her bill regardless of the source of payment.

Feel free to ask questions about your bill. Hospitals can and do make mistakes.

12. The patient has the right to know hospital rules and regulations that apply to his or her conduct as a patient.

A Patients Bill of Rights was reprinted with permission of the American Hospital Society, 1975.
(**ACCESS**PRESS LTD. comments printed here in italics).

RESPONSIBILITIES

50 What are my responsibilities?

You have a responsibility to:

Take care of yourself and participate in your plan of care. Ask questions, become involved in your care, verbalize your anxieties and fears. Let the staff know about your life. But most important, try to **make an effort to get better.**

Interact with the staff. Be sensitive to their workload, and try to address the right question to the right person.

Be a considerate roommate. Watch the noise level from your television, your conversations or your visitors. Do not smoke by the bedside of a non-smoker. Cooperate about the temperature of your room.

Communicate with your doctor. If you have a complaint or you feel that your treatment is not effective, question your doctor.

Read everything you sign. Even the simplest, most basic forms should be read. If you are groggy or nervous, ask your advocate to read your forms and help you ask questions.

51 How can I avoid making mistakes?

The best way to avoid any problems with your treatment is for you and your advocate to **ask questions.** Keep track of the answers to your questions and know what to expect. Ask everyone who is treating you (doctors, residents, nurses) what they are doing to and for you. **Ask for clarification if you do not understand.**

Remember to keep track of what tests you have had each day, medications, procedures, etc., in a log or journal. Your companion/advocate can help you. This will help you think of questions to ask and enable you to better **evaluate your bill** later when you leave the hospital. Even if you have a major medical policy that will cover almost all your expenses, there is no reason to be charged for blood that you did not receive or a procedure that was never performed. Mistakes can be made, and it is your responsibility to check your bill which will ultimately help **keep health care costs down.**

Discuss any lab work or tests that your doctor intends to order. **Be prepared** when a staff member comes to take you **for lab work,** and **make sure they have your correct name and orders.**

If you know that you are not supposed to eat solid foods or that you are not supposed to use salt, do not eat these items even if they come on your meal tray.

If you have been taking 1 white pill, every 4 hours, do not take the 3 pink ones that come in 2 hours without asking the nurse about them. Ask forcefully, and make sure that someone checks. Doctors, nurses and dieticians can make mistakes too. Never feel too intimidated to ask questions. It is **your health and your body. Know what is happening to it and why.**

52 What do I need to know about medication?

1. What is the **name** of the medication?
2. What is the **effectiveness** of this medication?
3. Are there any **adverse interactions** with food, vitamins or other drugs?
4. What are the **risks** of the medication?
5. What are the **side effects?**
6. Would the **side effects of another drug** be better or worse?
7. Ask if there are ways to **lessen the side effects** with another drug, diet or exercise.
8. If the medication is expensive, ask if there is a less expensive alternative or a **generic drug.** Generic drugs have the same quality as brand name drugs and may be less expensive. Prices vary from pharmacy to pharmacy.
9. How **long** will I have to take this medication?

For further information check **PDR: Physician's Desk Reference,** Medical Economic Company, 680 Kinderkamack Road, Oradell, NJ 07649.

53 How often am I allowed pain medicine?

The frequency and strength of pain medication varies from patient to patient depending on the type of procedure, your age, your overall health before the procedure and your tolerance for pain. Doctors have guidelines, but only you know how you are feeling. Find out the doctor's recommendations so you can ask for medication when you need it, but also realize that you should not ask for it more often than recommended. Usually pain medication will be prescribed **PRN (as needed)** but not more than every 4 hours. Your medication may take half an hour to start working. Therefore, ask for pain medication when you begin to feel uncomfortable rather than waiting until the pain is unbearable. It will take a stronger dose of pain medicine to alleviate the pain if you wait too long before asking.

54 What is a living will?

If you or someone else you know is critically ill, you might want to get a **living will.** While the patient is still alive, he or she can sign this will which directs the doctor and family not to use artificial procedures and devices, often referred to as **heroic measures,** to keep the patient alive. The form should be filed with a lawyer as well. The document will not always hold up in court, though some states endorse variations of the living will.

For information, contact **The Euthanasia Educational Council,** 250 W. 57 Street, New York, NY 10015, 212-246-6962.

As medical technology advances, doctors face the ethical, financial and legal questions of maintaining life with artificial devices daily. As health care costs rise, the financial question becomes more important.

If you want to request that life sustaining efforts not be made on your behalf, you must ask your physician to write this order on the medical chart, referred to as **No Code.** Otherwise, if an emergency situation arises, all life sustaining measures will be taken.

In a **New York Times/CBS News Poll**, *78 percent of the men and 77 percent of the women surveyed think doctors should stop using technical devices if the patient asks, even if that means the patient will die.*

Almost 28 percent of the nation's yearly Medicare budget goes toward maintaining people in their last years of life, and the bulk of that is spent during the last month of a patient's life.

HEALTH INFORMATION

55 What 8 ways can I get health information?

1. Start with a medical dictionary or general health care book:

Baby and Child Care
Dr. Benjamin Spock
Simon & Schuster
1230 Avenue of the Americas
New York NY 10020

The Patient's Advocate
Barbara Huffmann
Viking Press
(This book is out of print but try to find it at a public library.)

The Complete Health Care Advisor
Henry Berman MD and others
St. Martin's Press
175 Fifth Avenue
New York NY 10010

Medical Dictionary for the Non-Professional
Charles F. Chapman
Barron's Educational Series Inc.
113 Crossways Park Drive
Woodbury NY 11797

The American Medical Association Family Medical Guide
Jeffrey RM Kunz MD
Random House
201 E. 50 Street
New York NY 10022

2. **Health information centers** that are independently funded and provide unlimited public access to medical information. There are presently a few such centers in the country.

Boston Women's Health Collective
445 Mt. Auburn Street
Watertown MA 02172
617-924-0271

Center for Medical Consumers
237 Thompson Street
New York NY 10012
212-674-7105

Center for Consumer Health Education
1900 Association Drive
Reston VA 22091
703-476-3400

Consumer Health Information Center
East 600 South Street
Salt Lake City UT 84102
801-364-9318

Planetree Health Resource Center
2040 Webster Street
San Francisco CA 94115
415-923-3680

3. You can also get health information by **mail.** Planetree, a non-profit consumer oriented health group provides medical and health information by mail also. They will send you a **free mail order catalog** featuring over 60 self-care books and products. They can provide in-depth research packets on a wide range of topics. These packets consist of 30-35 pages of material gathered from current sources plus a computerized bibliography of medical literature. Some services require a small fee. For further information, contact **Planetree Health Resource Center**, 2040 Webster Street, San Francisco, CA 94115, 415-923-3680.

For information regarding hospitals or nursing homes, contact **American Hospital Association**, 840 N. Lake Shore Drive, Chicago, IL 60611, 312-280-6000.

4. **Self-help and support groups** can provide you with individual contacts who can lend a sympathetic ear and tell you of their own experience. For information or how to locate a nearby self-help group, contact **The Self-Help Center**, 1600 Dodge Avenue, Suite 122, Evanston, IL 60601, 312-328-0470.

5. **Health organizations** and agencies such as The American Cancer Society and American Diabetes Association can provide written literature, refer you to doctors and support groups and let you know about classes and lectures. Below is a list of the national headquarters of several health organizations.

American Cancer Society
777 Third Avenue
New York NY 10017
212-371-2900

American Diabetes Association
2 Park Avenue
New York NY 10016
212-683-7444

American Heart Association
7320 Greenville Avenue
Dallas TX 75231
214-750-5300

American Medical Association
535 N. Dearborn Street
Chicago IL 60610
312-751-6000

American Nurses Association
2420 Pershing Road
Kansas City MO 64108
816-474-5720

American Red Cross
17th & D Streets
NW Washington DC 20006
202-737-8300

6. **Hospitals and clinics** often sponsor lectures on a wide range of health topics from preventive medicine, such as workshops on health and fitness, to understanding and dealing with the emotional stress of a terminally ill family member.

7. **Public Libraries** are developing consumer health sections with current medical texts and lay books. You may be able to use the local university library, even if you are not a student. Many state supported school libraries have a mandate to provide open access.

8. **Hospital libraries** generally do not allow public use, but exceptions are sometimes made. Your physician may be able to authorize you to use the hospital library.

56 What medical or health publications are available?

1. There has been a proliferation of **health related newsletters and magazines** with current, objective, reliable health information. Some of the best popular periodicals include:

American Health
80 Fifth Avenue Suite 302
New York NY 10011

Harvard Medical School Health Letter
79 Garden Street
Cambridge MA 02138

Health Facts
Center For Medical Consumers
237 Thompson Street
New York NY 10012

Health Line
The Robert A. MacNeil Foundation
2855 Campus Drive
San Mateo CA 94403

Medical Self-Care Magazine
PO Box 717
Inverness CA 94937

2. Do not overlook **medical journals** written for physicians which have the most current information and are often written in clear, understandable language.

Journal of the American Medical Association (JAMA) (weekly)
535 N. Dearborn Street
Chicago IL 60610

Lancet (weekly)
Little Brown
34 Beacon Street
Boston MA 02106

Medical Tribune (weekly)
257 Park Avenue
New York NY 10010

New England Journal of Medicine (weekly)
10 Shattuck Street
Boston MA 01225

Post-graduate Medicine (monthly)
4530 W. 77th Street
Minneapolis MN 55435

3. **Government Sources.**

US Government Printing Office
(check your phone book for a local office)
Consumer Information Center
Public Documents Distribution
Pueblo CO 81009

National Health Information Clearinghouse
Box 1133
Washington DC 20013

Cancer Information Clearinghouse
7910 Woodmont Avenue Suite 1320
Bethesda MD 20014

Food and Drug Administration
Office of Consumer Affairs
5600 Fishers Lane (HFE-88)
Rockville MD 20857

HMO Trends

HMOs reduced hospitalization by 30 percent. Though HMOs attract a younger average population, studies with age standardization still found that HMO participants use fewer hospital days.

Participants in HMOs undergo one-half the amount of surgery as a population as a whole than non-participants.

There are 457/1000 days in the hospital for HMO participants compared to 822/1000 days for people covered by private insurance companies.

The average length of a hospital stay for HMO participants is 6.1 days while the average for people covered by private insurance companies is 7.4 days.

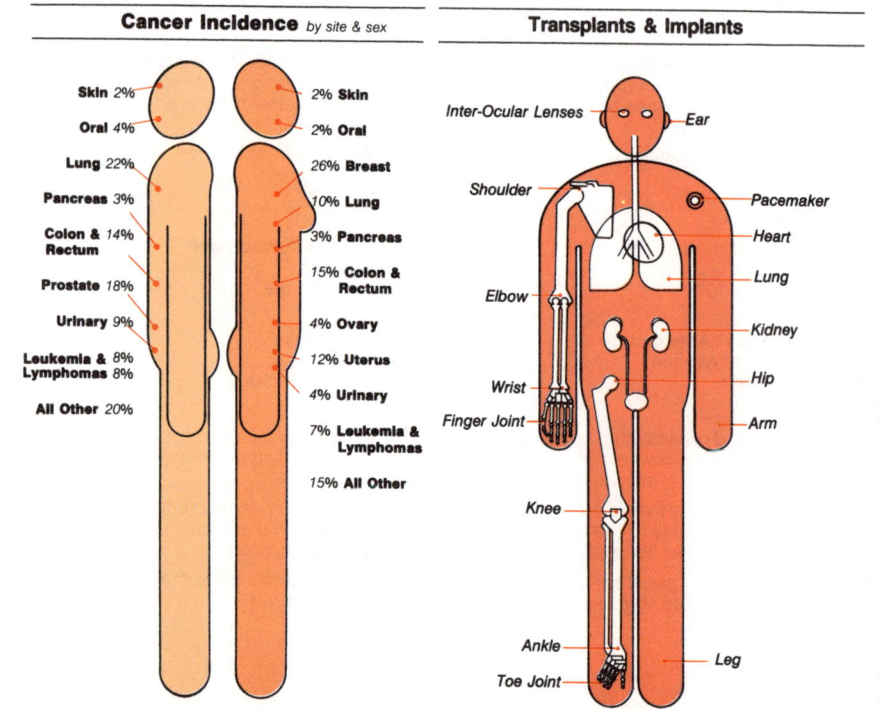

Cancer Incidence by site & sex

Male:
- Skin 2%
- Oral 4%
- Lung 22%
- Pancreas 3%
- Colon & Rectum 14%
- Prostate 18%
- Urinary 9%
- Leukemia & Lymphomas 8%
- All Other 20%

Female:
- 2% Skin
- 2% Oral
- 26% Breast
- 10% Lung
- 3% Pancreas
- 15% Colon & Rectum
- 4% Ovary
- 12% Uterus
- 4% Urinary
- 7% Leukemia & Lymphomas
- 15% All Other

Transplants & Implants

- Inter-Ocular Lenses
- Ear
- Shoulder
- Pacemaker
- Heart
- Elbow
- Lung
- Kidney
- Wrist
- Hip
- Finger Joint
- Arm
- Knee
- Ankle
- Leg
- Toe Joint

INSURANCE

57 *What do these insurance terms mean?*

The **UCR (Usual, Customary and Reasonable)** is the fee determined by your insurance company for a service based on the nature of that particular service and your geographic area. The insurance company then bases its payment on the UCR. Find out the UCR your company has established for the service you need, and compare it with the price that the doctor quotes you. There are 2 reasons for a discrepancy between the 2 fees. First, the insurance company may not be up-to-date. Second, the doctor may charge a fee higher than the usual one.

Calendar year refers to the period beginning on 1 January of any year and ending on 1 January of the following year.

Co-insurance is the percentage of your bill that you are required to pay for **covered expenses**. For example, if your policy has a $100 deductible with 20 percent co-insurance, you pay the $100 deductible and 20 percent of the covered expenses. You also pay for all services not covered by your policy. The insurance company pays the remaining 80 percent. Find out if there is a **ceiling** on the amount that you pay. For example, if the ceiling is $1000, the insurance company pays 100 percent of the remaining covered charges after you pay $1000.

Co-payment refers to the amount of the bill for which you are responsible. It is similar to a deductible but is only charged in **certain situations** such as an emergency room visit or for maternity charges.

The **deductible** is the amount you must pay before the insurance comes into effect. It is only applicable to services covered by your insurance policy. For example, if your policy does not cover routine physical exams, then you cannot use the fee you paid for a physical toward the deductible.

Physician Member is an **MD** or **DO** who contracts with your insurance company and agrees to accept the determined UCR, usually as part of a PPO.

58 *What should I know about insurance?*

Insurance policies vary greatly in what they cover and how much they cost. Because of the rising costs of health care, various alternatives, such as **Health Maintenance Organizations (HMOs)** and **Preferred Provider Organizations (PPOs)**, are being developed. The following is a list of 7 considerations for finding a good policy for you and/or your family.

1. Does the policy **cover accidents, illnesses** and **hospitalization?**

2. What **percent** of the bill is covered?

3. Does it offer **service benefits** (full coverage) or does it pay only on an **indemnity basis** which is a specified dollar amount per service?

4. What type of **deductible** is best for you?

5. When does **coverage take effect?**

6. Are there any **exclusionary clauses** which do not cover **pre-existing illnesses?**

7. What is the policy on **special items** such as **maternity, lab charges, prescription fees** or any other special concerns? Maternity coverage is often incomplete. Some policies cover the mother but not the baby unless the baby is sick. Others offer full coverage if you (the employee) get pregnant and virtually none if a male employee's wife gets pregnant.

Ask friends, relatives or coworkers about the company, just as you would when choosing a doctor or hospital. Ask other policy holders if the company answers claims quickly and courteously.

59 *What are the different types of coverage?*

A **Major Medical policy** covers catastrophic illnesses which may cost you thousands of dollars. Check to see if your current policy includes a major medical clause. If not, you may want to add one. Often, they are available at a fairly low rate.

Health Maintenance Organizations (HMOs) are a prepaid medical plan that offer a variety of health care services for a prepaid, fixed price. HMOs stress preventive care, early diagnosis and treatment on an outpatient basis. There are several different types of HMOs, depending on the source of funding and ownership. The desired qualities include **well-trained, board certified doctors,** a **system for doctors to review each other's work** and the **doctor/patient ratio should not exceed 1000 subscribers per primary care doctor.** For more information, contact:

Group Health Association of America
624 9th Street, Suite 700
Washington DC 20001

HMO Program
Department of HEW
Health Services Administration
6000 Fishers Lane
Rockville, MD 20852

HMO Toll Free Number
800-441-1910

Preferred Provider Organizations (PPOs) are another way to cut health care costs. In this situation, doctors and hospitals agree to provide participating businesses or individuals with health care services at a discounted rate. PPO is actually a **concept, not an actual organization or place.** Some of the common characteristics include:

1. A **discounted fee for service** for participants.

2. You can **receive care from a non PPO doctor,** but the reimbursement is lower.

3. Ways to **lower the level of utilization** and prevent over-utilization. Utilization is the term used to describe **the frequency with which physicians admit patients to the hospital.** In order to cut health care costs, PPOs try to avoid unnecessary hospitalization. However, if you are hospitalized by a PPO doctor, you will still receive coverage.

4. A simplified method of claims that enables **faster payment.**

5. Membership by a wide variety of physicians and hospitals to give patients **quality health care** and a **wide choice** in their physician.

Medicare, available for almost everyone 65 years-old and over and some disabled people under 65, **pays for some health care costs but does not cover everything.** Therefore, many people choose to purchase additional coverage, particularly a **major medical policy** to supplement their Medicare coverage and **guard against a longterm illness.** However, **beware of overinsuring.** Some companies will sell you duplicate coverage that Medicare already takes care of. Check with your local **Social Security office** for a full explanation of specifically what **Medicare** covers and when you need to sign up. Pick up a free copy of **Your Medicare Handbook** at your local Social Security office. Call them and they will mail you a copy.

Medicare is a 2-part health insurance program; **Part A covers hospital insurance** and **Part B covers medical insurance.** There are many regulations, conditions and exceptions. Contact your local **Social Security** office for advice on coverage for your particular illness or injury. Community centers or senior centers may be able to assist you also.

PART A—Hospital insurance helps you pay for 4 kinds of hospital care: **inpatient hospital care, medically necessary inpatient care in a skilled nursing facility after a hospital stay, home health care** and **hospice care.** A skilled nursing facility has specially qualified staff and equipment to provide skilled nursing care, rehabilitation services and other related health care. **Most nursing homes are not skilled nursing facilities.** Medicare will pay for most, but not all, of the services you receive in a hospital, skilled nursing facility or from a home health care agency or hospice program. Check which services are covered.

PART B—Medical insurance can help you pay for **doctors' services, outpatient hospital care, outpatient physical therapy, home health care** and some **health services and supplies** that are **not covered by Medicare hospital insurance.** Again, check **Your Medicare Handbook** for details.

The Medicare medical insurance currently has an initial **deductible** fee which means that you must pay the amount of the deductible before Medicare medical coverage begins. After you have paid the deductible, Medicare medical insurance covers 80 percent of your health care costs for covered services. You will have to pay for services that are not covered as well as 20 percent of the charge of covered services. Again, check **Your Medicare Handbook** available from your local social security office.

Medicaid pays medical bills for **low-income** people who cannot afford the costs of medical care. It is designed to **improve the health of people who might not have medical care** for themselves and their children.

Each state runs its own Medicaid program through a state welfare office, public health office, social service office or state Medicaid office. However, the **federal government pays approximately 55 percent of the nation's Medicaid bill.**

Medicaid currently covers medical services such as, **inpatient hospital service, outpatient hospital services, outpatient laboratory services such as x-rays** and **family planning services.** The services covered vary from state to state so check with your local office for details. You can also pick up a free booklet **Medicaid and You** from your local **Social Security office.**

Medicaid also provides special children's services called **EPSDT (early periodic screening diagnosis and treatment),** which **check general health** (nutrition, growth and development, vision), **detect diseases,** administer **immunization** programs and **diagnose** and **treat** problems before they result in permanent disability.

60 What are DRGs ?

A **Diagnosis Related Group (DRG)** is a way to categorize patients by the diagnosis of their condition. There are **23 major diagnostic categories (MDCs)** that are then further subdivided based on the patient's age and sex, the presence of any complications and the expected length of stay for each condition.

Congress has developed a pricing system to **reimburse hospitals for Medicare patients.** This **Prospective Payment System (PPS)** establishes a **fixed fee for medical services** based on each DRG (diagnosis related group). It is designed to reduce the skyrocketing cost of Medicare by lowering the fees for tests and procedures and encouraging shorter hospital stays.

Due to this system's apparent success in reducing costs, many **private insurance companies** are adopting the system as a means of reimbursing physicians for medical services, often through a PPO or an HMO.

Critics claim that the new system decreases the quality of health care because hospitals will be forced to release patients sooner than necessary in order to break even or make a profit. However, the **DRG category can be changed** if the patient's condition becomes worse as long as there is **appropriate documentation** to warrant a change. It will become increasingly important for nurses, patients' advocates and patients to be sure that accurate documentation about changes in a condition are **consistently recorded so that the DRG code is accurate.** The DRG system is the biggest change in health care since the establishment of Medicare that affects the entire country. The system is being closely monitored by the government and health care providers to determine its effectiveness.

MAJOR DIAGNOSTIC CATEGORIES

MDC 1 Diseases and Disorders of the Nervous System

MDC 2 Diseases and Disorders of the Eye

MDC 3 Diseases and Disorders of the Ear, Nose and Throat

MDC 4 Diseases and Disorders of the Respiratory System

MDC 5 Diseases and Disorders of the Circulatory System

MDC 6 Diseases and Disorders of the Digestive System

MDC 7 Diseases and Disorders of the Hepatobiliary System (Liver, Gall Bladder, Bile Ducts) and Pancreas

MDC 8 Diseases of the Musculoskeletal System and Corrective Tissue

MDC 9 Diseases of the Skin, Subcutaneous Tissue and Breast

MDC 10 Endocrine, Nutritional and Metabolic Diseases

MDC 11 Diseases and Disorders of the Kidney and Urinary Tract

MDC 12 Diseases and Disorders of the Male Reproductive System
MDC 13 Diseases and Disorders of the Female Reproductive System
MDC 14 Pregnancy, Childbirth and the Puerperium
MDC 15 Normal Newborns and Other Neonates with Certain Conditions Originating in the Perinatal Period
MDC 16 Diseases and Disorders of the Blood and Blood-forming Organs and Immunity
MDC 17 Myeloproliferative Disorders and Poorly Differentiated Malignancy (Cancer), Other Neoplasms NEC (Not elsewhere classified)
MDC 18 Infectious and Parasitic Diseases (Systemic)
MDC 19 Mental Disorders
MDC 20 Substance Use Disorders and Substance-induced Organic Disorders
MDC 21 Injury, Poisoning and Toxic Effects of Drugs
MDC 22 Burns
MDC 23 Selected Factors Influencing Health Status and Contact with Health Services

TOP 10 DRGs

1. **DRG 127** Heart failure and shock
2. **DRG 039** Lens Procedures
3. **DRG 182** Esophagitis, gastroenteritis and miscellaneous digestive disorders
4. **DRG 014** Simple cerebrovascular disorder (except transient ischemic attack)
5. **DRG 089** Simple pneumonia and pleurisy
6. **DRG 140** Angina pectoris
7. **DRG 088** Chronic obstructive pulmonary disease
8. **DRG 138** Cardiac dysrhythmias and conductive disorders
9. **DRG 243** Medical Back Problem
10. **DRG 096** Bronchitis and asthma

COSTS

61 *How can I reduce my hospital costs?*

Health care costs have been rising steadily and currently account for 11 percent of the GNP (gross national product). Some trends to reduce health care costs on a large scale include:

1. **Reduced compensation by Medicare** for certain procedures.

2. The implementation of **PPS (prospective payment system).**

3. The **transfer of payments** from private insurance companies to the beneficiary. It is easy to ignore health care costs if you are covered by a company policy which enables you to develop the attitude that someone else pays for medical bills. However, society as a whole pays for the skyrocketing increase in health care costs as insurance premiums increase to meet higher costs.

4. **Mandatory second opinion programs** to prevent unnecessary surgeries. One of the best ways to cut the cost of your hospital stay is to avoid it completely.

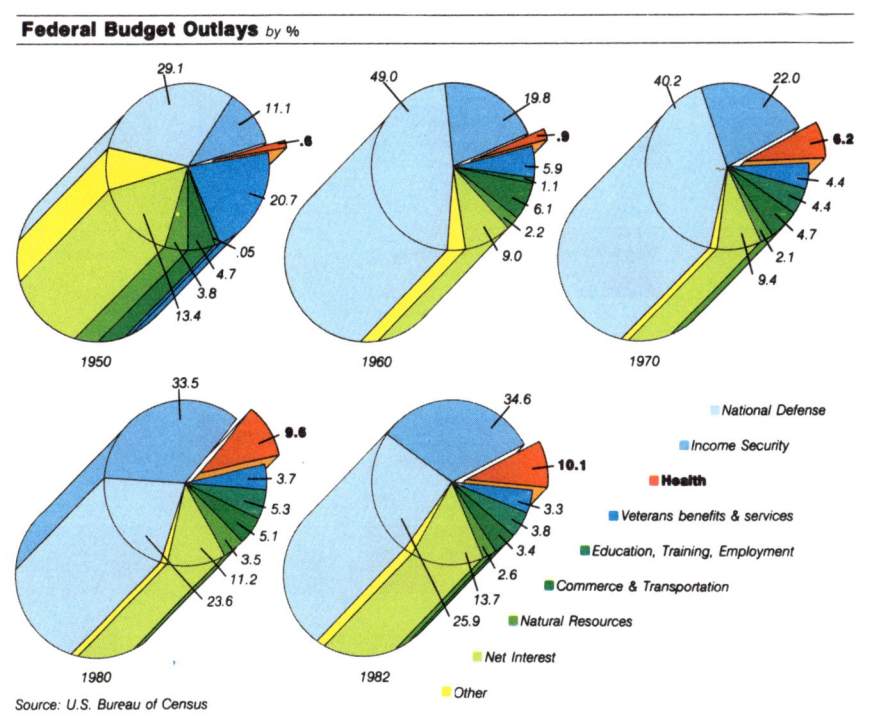

Federal Budget Outlays by %

Source: U.S. Bureau of Census

Most Frequent Operative Procedures
top ten for 1981 from short-stay hospitals

1. Biopsy
2. Dilation & Curettage
3. Excisions of lesions
4. Cesarean Section
5. Hysterectomy
6. Tubal Ligation
7. Extraction of Lens
8. Repair of Inguinal Hernia
9. Cholecystectomy
10. Oophorectomy

Source: 1983-84 Socio-Economic Factbook for Surgery

Ambulatory Surgery Procedures
top ten for 1981

1. Dilation & Curettage
2. Laparoscopy
3. Orthopedic procedures
4. Myringotomy (removal of eardrum)
5. Excision of mass/skin lesion
6. Arthroscopy
7. Tonsillectomy and/or adenoidectomy
8. Dental procedures
9. Plastic procedures
10. Cystoscopy

Source: Freestanding Ambulatory Surgical Association 1982

Malpractice *Cause & Effect*

According to New York Magazine, 18 March 1985, the 4 most common reasons for malpractice are:
1. Incorrect or late diagnosis
2. Alleged mishandling of pregnancy, labor and delivery that leads to neurological problems
3. Surgical complications
4. Lack of informed consent

The 3 specialties with the highest number of claims filed against them are neurosurgery, orthopedics and OB/GYN according to New York Magazine 18 March 1985.

One of the most common reasons for malpractice suits is that patients believe that physicians do not make mistakes.

Because of the increase in malpractice suits and the cost of malpractice insurance, many doctors have had to change their attitudes and are more conscious of defensive medicine. Defensive medicine translates to higher costs:
1. In order to protect themselves, physicians perform more diagnostic tests and lab work to rule out a wider variety of possibilities.
2. Some doctors are refusing to perform high risk surgery.
3. Physicians must decide whether to make their patients feel safe and secure or warn them of a possible complication even if it only occurs 2-3 percent of the time.

Physician Visits *per person / by family income*

1981 Income	Visits
Less than $7,000	5.6
$7,000-$9,999	4.9
$10,000-$14,999	4.5
$15,000-$24,999	4.5
$25,000 And up	4.4

Life Expectancy at Birth

Year	Male	Female
1978	69.6	77.3
1979	70.0	77.8
1980	70.0	77.5
1981	70.3	77.9
1982	70.8	78.2

Three Leading Causes of Death *United States / by age & sex*

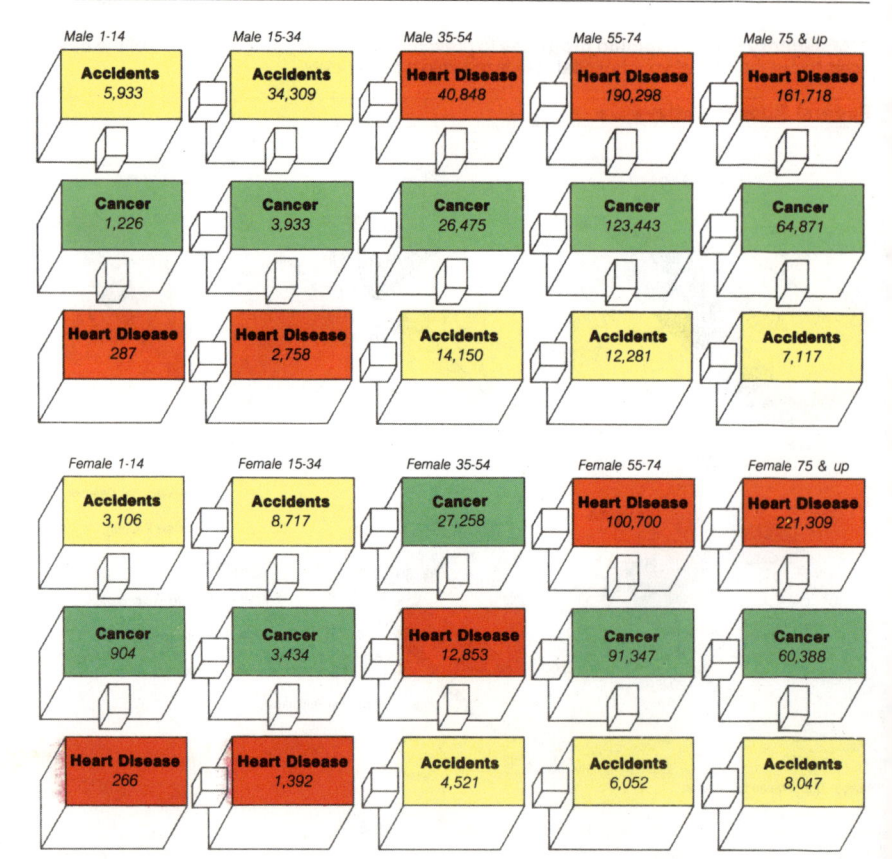

Male 1-14
- Accidents 5,933
- Cancer 1,226
- Heart Disease 287

Male 15-34
- Accidents 34,309
- Cancer 3,933
- Heart Disease 2,758

Male 35-54
- Heart Disease 40,848
- Cancer 26,475
- Accidents 14,150

Male 55-74
- Heart Disease 190,298
- Cancer 123,443
- Accidents 12,281

Male 75 & up
- Heart Disease 161,718
- Cancer 64,871
- Accidents 7,117

Female 1-14
- Accidents 3,106
- Cancer 904
- Heart Disease 266

Female 15-34
- Accidents 8,717
- Cancer 3,434
- Heart Disease 1,392

Female 35-54
- Cancer 27,258
- Heart Disease 12,853
- Accidents 4,521

Female 55-74
- Heart Disease 100,700
- Cancer 91,347
- Accidents 6,052

Female 75 & up
- Heart Disease 221,309
- Cancer 60,388
- Accidents 8,047

5. The development of **HMOs and PPOs**

As an individual patient, some of the ways to **reduce the cost of your hospital stay** include:

1. Ask your doctor if you need to be in the hospital the night before your surgery. You can **save one day's cost by coming to the hospital early on the day of your surgery.** If you need to be at the hospital the night before, **check in late and check out early.** Like hotels, hospitals have a specific time when the admission day begins and ends.

2. Ask about **telephone and television charges.** Keep your in-room telephone calls to a minimum because they will cost more than calls from home. If you need to talk to people, call and ask them to call you right back.

3. **Question any procedure** that you think is **unnecessary, especially lab work and diagnostic tests.** Try to have any pre-admission tests done before checking into the hospital. You may be able to have them performed at the doctor's office.

4. Talk to your doctor about **going home as early as you feel comfortable.**

5. Ask if **home care** is available.

6. **Avoid buying items from the hospital** like hand lotion, toothpaste or shampoo. You will pay more than at a supermarket. Ask your advocate or companion to purchase what you need outside of the hospital.

7. If you are continuing to take medications that you have already purchased, you may get permission from your doctor to bring in your own drugs. However, the doctor must write on your chart, **patient may take own medication.** Drugs purchased through the hospital pharmacy tend to be more expensive.

62 When can I leave the hospital?

Technically, you can leave the hospital any time that you would like though it may be **against medical advice.** Your insurance may not cover any part of your stay if you leave against medical advice. Check before making a decision. Otherwise, your physician will decide when you can return home. Ask your doctor, nurse, or someone in the hospital's Social Service Department about special equipment or nursing care you will need and where to get it. For elderly patients, check if you are eligible for visiting nursing care through Medicare.

Be sure you **know which medication** to take and why to take it. Get a complete rundown on your **activities** and **future appointments.** If you are discharged with **special diet instructions** such as soft food, low sodium or a bland diet, ask your physician for diet guidelines. Be sure that your doctor informs you of all the **exercises** you must do and **know how to do them.** Find out when you can **return to your regular activities.** Depending on the nature of your surgery, you may have limited mobility during the first few weeks out of the hospital. What once seemed like simple activities may make you very tired or weak at first.

63 Do I see my bill before I leave?

You or your advocate or companion should see your bill before you leave. **Check that all the information is correct.** Some of it may be difficult to decipher. For example, the tests and procedures may be in technical terms. If you have any questions, ask your doctor, nurse or patient's representative.

As mentioned earlier, you should keep a journal or log of all the tests, procedures, lab work or any other special services that you receive.

EMERGENCIES

64 How can I prepare for an emergency?

Not all hospitals have emergency rooms, and some emergency rooms are better than others. **Shop around for the best emergency room in your area.** Start with the hospital where your family doctor has admitting privileges. **Proximity to your home** is also important. In an emergency, you do not want to have to go cross-town. Find the easiest route by car or public transportation.

Get a map of your community. Post it where all family members can find it. **Indicate emergency spots,** such as **hospitals, your doctors' offices, police and fire departments** and **burn and trauma centers.**

Post a list of phone numbers for:

1. police and fire departments
2. ambulances
3. paramedics
4. burn and trauma centers
5. your family doctor
6. nearest relative or neighbor in case your children are alone or with a babysitter.

65 What are emergency rooms, trauma centers and urgent care centers?

Hospital Emergency Rooms (ERs) fall into 2 categories: stand-by and 24-hour. Most hospitals have 24-hour ERs which require an emergency room physician to be present 24 hours a day. Most 24-hour ERs have specialists on call within half an hour. **Paramedics and ambulances are required to take the victim to the nearest 24-hour ER.** Stand-by ERs do not have a physician present 24 hours a day but there is a nurse on duty.

Trauma Centers are special units within a 24-hour ER that only treat severe trauma patients requiring surgical intervention within an hour, often referred to as *the golden hour.* Ninety-nine percent of the patients treated in a trauma center are brought in by paramedics. A **trauma team,** including a surgeon, an anesthesiologist, (and often specialists such as a neurosurgeon) are on duty 24 hours a day. At least one operating room suite is reserved for their use.

However, the presence of a trauma center does not mean that the quality of the care is better within the ER itself. You cannot choose to use the trauma center; that is a medical decision based on your condition.

Urgent Care or **Emergi Centers** are freestanding facilities that are not affiliated with a hospital. They are often less expensive because they do not have the overhead costs of a hospital ER. Urgent Care or Emergi Centers can **provide minor emergency care** but they lack the back-up resources of a hospital emergency room. They can treat problems such as splints, minor stitches for deep cuts or minor burns.

However, if you have a life-threatening situation such as severe chest pains or an undiagnosed problem like high fever or convulsions, go directly to the hospital because it is better equipped to analyze and treat you.

66 What is considered an emergency?

Most doctors consider any of the following an emergency:

- severe and uncontrollable bleeding
- poisoning
- choking
- shortness of breath or difficulty breathing
- insect stings resulting in shortness of breath
- convulsions
- severe burns (heat or chemical)
- bullet or stab wounds
- unconsciousness
- overdose of drugs
- severe chest pains
- eye injuries or foreign substance in the eye or sudden loss of vision
- heat stroke/dehydration
- hypothermia (dangerously low body temperature)
- broken bones
- head injury
- smoke inhalation
- inhalation of gaseous fumes
- severe abdominal pain
- slurring or loss of speech
- temperature over 103 degrees
- prolonged vomiting or diarrhea
- snake or animal bites

When in doubt, call the ER or your doctor. They are available to serve your needs and to help you avoid more serious problems.

Check if there is a children's hospital in your neighborhood. They will be better prepared to care for infants and small children because they specialize in children's injuries and diseases. If there is not one close by, a regular ER is prepared to care for children in an emergency.

It is recommended to **keep a signed emergency consent form** with your children or babysitter in case you cannot be reached in an emergency situation. Check with the ER where you are most likely to go for a specific form for that hospital. Or, **keep a letter** that gives permission **for a third party to give consent** if the situation warrants it.

67 What is 911 emergency service?

This service enables the caller to dial **9-1-1** for any emergency situation, such as fire, heart attack or robbery. The service features **automatic call location** so the call can be directed to the nearest ambulance, fire or police department.

Approximately 45 percent of the country is covered by a form of centralized emergency service. It is a federally encouraged program, but it is privately funded and operated by the telephone companies. There is often a small surcharge on your monthly phone bill to support the service.

If **911 is not available** in your community, **learn the numbers of the police and fire departments.**

68 What will the dispatcher need to know?

1. The **victim's address and phone number** and any special directions. After dark, be sure the home or emergency site is well lit so the emergency vehicle can locate you.

2. A brief, **coherent description of the problem,** including age and sex of the patient. For example, my 3 year-old son fell off the swing set and is lying unconscious in the backyard, or my 70 year-old mother slipped on the ice on the front porch and is unable to move her left leg and has difficulty moving her left arm. We have wrapped her in blankets to keep her warm but are unable to move her into the house.

3. Your name.

4. **Do not hang-up.** The dispatcher may need additional information.

Call the patient's doctor for advice or to meet you. If your doctor is at the ER, he or she can speed up the waiting process and treat you or have you admitted directly into the hospital. **If there is not time to call your doctor, the emergency vehicle is equipped with communications equipment** and keeps in close contact with the hospital personnel so they are ready for your arrival. The emergency vehicle personnel can also get a call to your doctor.

69 Do I need to bring anything to the ER?

Yes. Bring information regarding **your insurance policy.** Your insurance company should give you a card to keep in your wallet with your **policy number** on it. Without insurance information, the hospital may make you pay on the spot. If a patient does not have insurance or cannot pay immediately, hospitals must evaluate and stabilize an emergency. However, the case is usually transferred to a tax supported community hospital.

If the problem involves **poisoning** or a **drug overdose, bring the container** to the emergency room. Also bring any medication that you take regularly.

70 What should I do if a severe situation arises that is not an emergency?

Call your family physician. If the doctor is with a patient, it may take half an hour or so for someone to get back to you. If you are not calling during office hours, find out if your doctor is on call or if another doctor in the office is on call. The doctor may make arrangements to meet you at the office or at the ER, or he or she may refer you to a specialist, depending on the nature of the problem.

For example, if your child falls off a swingset onto his or her wrist, the pediatrician may want the wrist examined by an orthopedic surgeon.

71 What happens if I go to the emergency room for a non-emergency problem?

You will have **to wait,** and it will **cost more** than a clinic or visit to your primary care physician. ERs are for emergencies and **patients are treated in the order of severity.** The priorities of an emergency room are:

1. **Save lives immediately endangered,** such as shock as the result of an accident, heart attack or severe bleeding.

2. **Uncover and treat illnesses or injuries that might become life threatening** within minutes or hours, such as severe abdominal pains that may become appendicitis or a head injury that may have resulted in internal bleeding.

3. **Manage emergency problems,** such as broken bones or severe vomiting caused by stomach virus, **that are not life threatening** but require treatment and relief from pain and suffering. Use your doctor or outpatient clinic for minor or chronic problems.

72 What first-aid procedures should I know?

Learn cardio-pulminary resuscitation (CPR), the **Heimlich maneuver** and **basic first-aid** that teaches how to stop severe bleeding and how to induce vomiting for some types of poisoning. Many local hospitals and organizations, such as the fire department, local colleges or the YMCA/YWCA provide courses. Contact your local American Heart Association and American Red Cross offices for information regarding classes or contact the national office for information: **American Heart Association**, 7320 Greenville Ave, Dallas, TX 75231, 214-750-5300 or **American Red Cross**, 17th & D Streets NW, Washington DC, 20006, 202-737-8300.

If a victim stops breathing and/or you cannot detect a heart beat by taking a pulse at the **Carotid Artery** on either side of the throat, you may be able to save a life by using the techniques learned in a **CPR course.** Only 4-6 minutes can elapse before loss of oxygen causes permanent brain damage or death. Many medical authorities agree that everyone over 13 years old should learn CPR.

For a quick reference for first-aid procedures, check the first section of your local phone book. For more detailed information, check **The Family First Aid & Medical Guide,** Dr. James Bevan, Simon & Schuster, 1230 Avenue of the Americas, New York, NY 10020.

73 What precautions should I take if I have a chronic illness or allergies to medicine?

Keep the name of your physician and telephone number, your hospital of preference and the names of persons to be notified in an emergency in your wallet.

Medic Alert tags should be worn by people with chronic illnesses, such as diabetes or epilepsy or if you are allergic to any medication, such as penicillin or codeine. **Your medical condition, membership number** and a **24-hour phone number** that provides instant access to your medical records and the name and number of physicians and relatives to contact are located on the back of your tag. You can also obtain **wallet-sized cards on microfilm** that contain your health information and a wallet-sized magnifying glass to read the card. If you are **unconscious, stunned or confused due to an accident,** attending personnel such as paramedics or emergency room doctors, know to take special precautions in treating you.

You can only purchase a Medic Alert tag through the **Medic Alert Foundation,** PO Box 1009, Turlock, CA 95381, 800-344-3226 or 800-468-1020 (in California).

For information regarding the microfilm cards contact **National Health and Safety Awareness Center,** Application Department Suite 927, 333 N. Michigan Avenue, Chicago, IL 60601, 312-726-6499.

74 How do I get health care overseas?

Health care problems while traveling abroad can become a nightmarish experience with unnecessary complications. With a little planning, you can avoid difficulty in obtaining health care abroad.
International Association for Medical Assistance to Travelers (IAMAT), 736 Center Street, Lewiston, NY 14092, 716-754-4883 and **Intermedic Inc.,** 777 Third Avenue, New York, NY 10017, 212-486-8974 can provide you with more information.

IAMAT has no membership fee and provides you with a directory of member doctors serving in over 450 cities. The doctors, educated in international medical practices, all speak English.

Their services are available 24 hours a day and the fee depends on whether you make an office visit or the doctor makes a hotel or house call. Membership also entitles you to the **Travelers Clinical Record** which should be filled out by your physician and carried with you on all your travels, both domestic and abroad. You also receive the **World Immunization and Malaria Risk Chart** which describes each country's immunization laws and the malaria risk, if any. Be sure to take care of immunization well in advance of your scheduled departure.

For a small yearly membership fee, **Intermedic** provides you with a list of English-speaking doctors throughout the world whose fees depend on whether you visit the office or if the doctor makes a house or hotel call. They can also provide you with information concerning immunization and malaria.

If you are in a city that is not listed by either of these organizations, contact the American Embassy for a list of local English-speaking doctors.

ABBREVIATIONS

a. c. before meals
AMA American Medical Association
b. i. d. twice a day
bib drink
BP blood pressure
BRP bathroom privileges
Bx biopsy
c̄ with
CAD coronary artery disease
CBC complete blood count
CC chief complaint
CCU coronary care unit
chol. cholesterol
CPR Cardio Pulminary Resuscitation
cxr chest x-ray
D & C dilation and curettage
DRG diagnosis related groups
Dx diagnosis
ECG or EKG electrocardiogram
EEG electroencephalogram
EENT eyes, ears, nose & throat
ER emergency room
FH family history
GI gastrointestinal
GP general practitioner
GYN gynecology
HMO health maintenance organization
HPI history present illness
hs at bedtime
Hx history
ICU intensive care unit
IV intravenous
JCAH Joint Commission on Accreditation of Hospitals
LPN licensed practical nurse
LVN licensed vocational nurse
Na low sodium
NPO nothing by mouth
OOB out of bed
OR operating room
PH past history
PI previous illness
pc after meals
PPO preferred provider organization

PRN as needed
PT physical therapy
px prognosis
q. every
q. d. every day
q. h. every hour
q. i. d. four times a day
RBC red blood cell
RN registered nurse
Rx prescription
s̄ without
T & A tonsillectomy & adenoidectomy
Tb tuberculosis
t.i.d three times a day
TPR temperature, pulse, respiration
VS vital signs
WBC white blood count

COMMON MEDICAL PREFIXES
(usually describe time or place)

a- without
adeno- glandular
amphi- both sides
ante- before
anti- against
bi- two, twice, double
circum- around
dia- through, across
dys- difficult
ecto- outside
endo- inside
hemi- half
hyper- over, excessive, above
hypo- under, deficient
infra- underneath, below
inter- among, between
intra- within
iso- equal
mal- disordered
meta- after or changing
post- after
pre- before
retro- backward
sub- under
super- over
supra- above

SUFFIXES (Usually denote an act or condition)

-algia pain
-asis condition
-cide killer
-dynia pain
-ectomy cut out, surgical removal
-emia blood
-genesis production, development
-iatrist specialist
-iatry field of medicine
-itis inflammation
-logy study of
-oma tumor
-oscopy viewing an organ
-osis condition
-pathy disease, abnormality
-penia abnormal reduction
-pexy fix or sew in place
-phasia speaking condition
-plasty to restore or reconstruct
-ptosis falling, downward displacement
-rrhea flow or discharge
-scope instrument for examination
-stomy creation of an opening
-uria urine

ROOTS (parts of the body)

adeno gland
arthro joint
cardio heart
chole gall
cholecyst gall bladder
col colon
colpo vagina
crania skull
cysto bladder
dermia, dermato skin
entero intestines
gastro stomach
hema,
hemo,
hemato blood
hepato liver
hystero uterus

Richard Saul Wurman

Michael Everitt *Project Director*

Editorial & Writing
Digby Diehl
Kay Diehl
Jonathan Shestack *Tests*
Jean Carroll *Surgery*
Abbe Don *Questions & Answers*
Eileen Yamada

Margaret Jones
Paula Van Gelder
Linda Lenhoff
Gretel Goldsmith

Design Surgery
Peter Bradford
Lorraine Johnson

Design & Production
Warren Nung
Hugh Enockson
Tom Wood
Brian Sisco
Rebecca Chamlee Keeley
Sue Pace

Typesetting
Robin Carr
George Quioan
Jack Skelley

Research
Ellen Lupton
Eileen O'Neill
Sara Lukinson
Devorah Rosen

Proofreading
Luisa Lorona

Administrative Support
Randy Walburger
Carrie Enoch
Chris Toronto

Cover Photo
Reven T.C. Wurman

Printing
McGill-Jensen
Bill Dorich

Photocomposition
McGill-Jensen

Special Thanks
American Medical International
National Medical Advisory
Council of AMI
for overall review of text

Planetree Health Resource Center
Patricia Phelan
Founding Executive Director
Rochelle Perrine Schmalz
Resource Center Director
for research and review of text

Bobrow Thomas & Associates
Architects, Planners, Consultants
for research on OR and ICU diagrams

Thanks:
Arthur Sackler MD
William Wolgin MD
Jack M. Matloff MD
Daniel Kanofsky MD
Barry Mennen MD

Special Thanks to **Peter Bradford** and his **staff** for extraordinary work on the surgery section of this book.

Richard Saul Wurman, FAIA, is an architect, graphic designer, cartographer and recipient of Guggenheim, Graham, Chandler, Annenberg and NEA Fellowships. He has authored, co-authored and designed more than 35 publications including: **Urban Atlas, Making the City Observable, Cities: Comparison of Form and Scale, Man-Made Philadelphia, Various Dwellings Described in a Comparative Manner, Yellow Pages of Learning Resources, Yellow Pages Career Library, The Nature of Recreation, Notebooks and Drawings of Louis I. Kahn, Whole Pacific Catalog.** Mr. Wurman served as a member of the policy panel for the National Endowment for the Arts, Design Arts Program, Chairman of the 1972 IDCA Conference, Co-Chairman of the 1st Federal Design Assembly, 1973, Co-Chairman of T.E.D., The Technology Entertainment Design Communications Conference, 1984, and has many university affiliations, currently University Fellow of the New School For Social Research, NYC. He is a board member of the American Institute of Graphic Arts.

ACCESSPRESS Ltd.
Richard Saul Wurman
Frank Stanton
Co-owners

ACCESSPRESS publications are distributed by
Simon & Schuster, Inc.
1230 Avenue of the Americas
New York NY 10020

Toll Free Number for orders:
1-800-223-2336

In NY State   In NYC
(excluding NYC)   757-9152
1-800-442-7070